ENVIRONMENTAL TOXICOLOGY:
THE LEGACY OF *SILENT SPRING*

The transcript of a Witness Seminar held by the Wellcome Trust Centre
for the History of Medicine at UCL, London, London, on 12 March 2002

Edited by D A Christie and E M Tansey

Volume **19** 2004

CONTENTS

Introduction
John Clark
v

Acknowledgements
xi

Witness Seminars: Meetings and publications
xiii
E M Tansey and D A Christie

Transcript
Edited by D A Christie and E M Tansey
1

References
75

Biographical notes
89

Glossary
95

Index
99

INTRODUCTION

As she struggled against ill-health to complete her fourth and final book, Rachel Carson pondered the best course of treatment for her cancer: chemicals or radiation.[1] Described as one of the most important contributions to Western literature and as one of the 'books that changed America',[2] *Silent Spring* (1962) is also considered the 'effective beginning' of 'toxic discourse'.[3] Radiation and chemicals linger in the text of *Silent Spring*. Drawing the reader's attention to these twin toxic hazards, Carson effectively fused the pre-existent pollution concerns of urban and industrial reformers to the ecological sensitivities of resource conservation and wilderness preservation. Her forceful vision helped to establish the modern environmental movement.[4] Forty years after the publication of *Silent Spring*, the Wellcome Trust Centre's Witness Seminar convened to assess the legacy of this book in relation to environmental toxicology.

As a belief that disease or illness might be determined by physical surroundings, 'environmentalism' had roots in antiquity. But the second half of the seventeenth century witnessed a revival of Hippocratic teaching that connected disease to airs, waters and places. Beginning in the late eighteenth century, a contingent of Edinburgh-trained medical practitioners drew upon this revival to locate medical problems in a wider social context. They linked disease to overcrowding, and to a lack of cleanliness and ventilation. By the 1830s, this activist, 'environmentalist' medicine had become subsumed within Chadwickian social reform (page 49).[5]

By the twentieth century, however, changes in theories of disease causation and in the organization of medicine effected a reassessment of the relationship between physical environment and human health and disease. The twentieth

---

[1] Lear L. (1997) *Rachel Carson: Witness for nature*. London: Penguin Books, 378–9.

[2] Lutts R H. (1985) Chemical Fallout: Rachel Carson's *Silent Spring* [Carson R. (1962)], radioactive fallout and the environmental movement. *Environmental Review* 9: 211–25, 211.

[3] Buell L. (2001) *Writing for an Endangered World: Literature, culture, and environment in the US and beyond*. Cambridge (USA) and London: The Belknap Press, 35.

[4] See Walker M J. (1999) The unquiet voice of *Silent Spring*. The legacy of Rachel Carson. *The Ecologist* 29: 322–5.

[5] See Flinn M W. (1965) Introduction to Edwin Chadwick *The Sanitary Condition of the Labouring Population of Great Britain*. Edinburgh: Edinburgh University Press, 1–73; Riley J. C. (1987) *The Eighteenth-century Campaign to Avoid Disease*. Basingstoke: Macmillan; Hamlin C. (1998) *Public Health and Social Justice in the Age of Chadwick, 1800–1854*. Cambridge: Cambridge University Press.

century ushered in an 'epidemiological transition' from a pre-industrial demographic regime, dominated by epidemic infectious diseases, to modern patterns of death from chronic degenerative diseases. At the same time, the rise of scientific medicine generated an elevated awareness of disease and illness.[6] Written under the pseudonym Lewis Herber, Murray Bookchin's *Our Synthetic Environment* placed this epidemiological transition in the post-Second World War context. Published in the same year as *Silent Spring*, Bookchin's book argued that concerns for infectious diseases had been replaced by environmentally related public health problems, such as heart disease and cancer (pages 19 and 25).[7]

As Carson pointed out, the synthetic insecticide industry was 'a child of the Second World War'.[8] Although the insecticidal properties of DDT were discovered by Paul Müller just prior to the outbreak of hostilities in 1939, the Second World War provided this new chlorinated hydrocarbon insecticide with the perfect stage on which to showcase its properties (page 4). Wartime concerns for agricultural production and for the threat of insect vectors of disease helped to accelerate the dispersal and acceptance of DDT. Faced with a post-war industrial cache of the insecticide, the US government released DDT for civilian use in August 1945, before the completion of definitive tests for chronic toxicity. Within less than a decade, the total USA production of DDT rose from approximately 10 million pounds to over 100 million pounds in 1951. By the time that Carson drew attention to the pervasive presence of this insecticide, US production had peaked at 188 million pounds. And its success spawned the introduction of 25 new pesticides.[9]

The knowledge and application of insecticides were not new: they had an ancient ancestry. Most often meant for small-scale household and garden applications, a variety of organic materials had been employed. The use of animal and vegetable oils and tars stretched back to antiquity. From the late seventeenth century, tobacco, hellebore, quassia, derris, pyrethrum, soap, and lime all became

---

[6] Weindling P. (1992) From infectious to chronic diseases: Changing patterns of sickness in the nineteenth and twentieth centuries, in Wear A. (ed.) *Medicine in Society: Historical essays.* Cambridge: Cambridge University Press, 303–16.

[7] See Gottlieb R. (1993) *Forcing the Spring: The transformation of the American environmental movement.* Washington: Island Press, 87.

[8] Carson R. (1962; rept. 1987) *Silent Spring.* Boston: Houghton Mifflin, 16.

[9] See Perkins J H. (1978) Reshaping technology in wartime: The effect of military goals on entomological research and insect-control practices. *Technology and Culture* 19: 169–86; Lear L. (1997): 119.

recognized pest control substances. But the late nineteenth century witnessed the first mass application of inorganic toxic insecticides (pages 3–4). The ravages of the Colorado beetle, the gypsy moth, and the cotton boll weevil evoked the introduction of the best-known arsenical insecticides – Paris green, lead arsenate and calcium arsenate. Although perfectly aware of the poisonous attributes of these insecticides, medical opinion most often focused on acute toxicity and neglected chronic toxicity.[10] In the wake of the epidemiological transition, Carson reversed this focus. But it was not simply the shift from acute infectious to chronic degenerative diseases that provided *Silent Spring* with fertile ground for its warnings of the 'pollution of the total environment of mankind'.[11]

Highly visible fatal pollution events had certainly highlighted the urban industrial threat to public health prior to the publication of *Silent Spring*. Killer smogs in the Meuse valley, Belgium (1930), Donora, Pennsylvania (1948), and London (1952) (pages 38 and 52) demonstrated the lethal cost of the twentieth century's unprecedented consumption of fossil fuels.[12] But Carson alerted the public to an invisible pollutant that could travel great distances, accumulate in body fats, and cause cancer, birth defects and mutations. *Silent Spring* was a child of the Cold War. Explicitly pairing chemical insecticides with radiation, Carson wrote in the shadow of the apocalyptic mushroom clouds over Hiroshima and Nagasaki.[13] Moreover, by noting the close relationship between insecticides and chemical warfare, she cast these substances in the nefarious role of weapons of war and mass destruction (pages 4 and 33).[14]

Silent Spring opened with 'a fable for tomorrow'. It described a community bereft of the beauty of wildflowers: in which fruit trees were barren, birds silenced, and 'everywhere was a shadow of death…No witchcraft, no enemy action had silenced the rebirth of new life in this stricken world. The people had done it

---

[10] See Whorton J. (1974); Clark J F M. (2001) Bugs in the system: Insects, agricultural science, and professional aspirations in Britain, 1890–1920. *Agricultural History* 75: 83–114.

[11] Carson R. (1962; rept. 1987): 39.

[12] See Brimblecombe P. (1987). For an excellent account of the historically unprecedented scale and pace of anthropogenic environmental change in the twentieth century, see McNeill J. (2000) *Something New Under the Sun: An environmental history of the twentieth-century world.* London: Allen Lane.

[13] This is essentially the point made by Lutts R H. (1985).

[14] Carson R. (1962; rept. 1987): 16. In addition, see Russell E. (2001); Weindling P J. (2000) *Epidemics and Genocide in Eastern Europe, 1890–1945.* Oxford: Oxford University Press, for the relationships between insecticides and chemical and biological warfare.

themselves'.[15] Although genetic and other ecological 'mega-hazards' have been added to nuclear and chemical threats, the fable for tomorrow retains its resonance as a powerful allegory of the 'Risk Society'. Post-industrial society struggles collectively to come to terms with the indeterminate risks to human survival that have been forged on the glowing embers of a faith in progress. Unlike the famines, epidemics and natural catastrophes that haunted pre-industrial society, these new hazards have been generated by human decisions. Paradoxically, much of the collective anxiety stems from an inability to determine with any precision the extent of the threat (pages 11–12, 20, 23).[16] Environmental epidemiology, for instance, can rarely identify exposure to a specific chemical at a particular time as the cause of a single person's disease (pages 47–8, 66–70). Moreover, arguments rage over who should determine the nature of a risk. As the authors of many of the hazards, technocrats may not be the most suitable choices. In an effort to establish a guide for potentially harmful human activities, a group of individuals met at Wingspread in Racine, Wisconsin, in January 1998. They agreed that where large numbers of humans were faced with potentially irreversible harm, it was best to err on the side of caution: they produced a statement on the 'precautionary principle'[17] (pages 16, 20, 24, 72).

Perhaps shaped by the limitations imposed by her gender, Rachel Carson forged a career in science that placed her in an ideal position to offer a timely critique of the technocratic society. From a very early age, she honed her talents as both a naturalist and a writer. While pursuing her undergraduate degree at the Pennsylvania College for Women, she vacillated between English and science before finally opting for a major in the latter. And after graduating from Johns Hopkins University with a Master's degree in zoology, she enjoyed a successful career as a writer and editor for the Bureau of US Fisheries (which later became the US Fish and Wildlife Service). After almost 16 years at this job, and after the publication of three popular books on marine biology, Carson had the scientific knowledge and a vast network of expert friends, colleagues and acquaintances upon which she could draw for the production of her final, and most controversial, book.[18]

---

[15] Carson R. (1962; rept. 1987): 1–3.

[16] Beck U. (1992) From industrial society to the risk society: Questions for survival, social structure and ecological enlightenment. *Theory, Culture & Society* 9: 97–123.

[17] Montague P. (1998). The precautionary principle. *Rachel's Environment & Health Weekly*, no. 586, February 19. See www.psrast.org/precaut.htm (site accessed 13 April 2004).

[18] See Lear L. (1997) for an excellent biographical account.

As a warning of the hazards of industrial pollutants, *Silent Spring* was born of important changes to the countryside. Post-war reconstruction entailed an intensification of agricultural production that accelerated in the years following 1960 (page 6). Farming metamorphosed into 'agribusiness' as holdings increased; specialization and mechanization flourished as the mixed farm went into sharp decline. Cheap nitrogenous fertilizers were applied to enhance soil fertility (page 21) and a 'huge expansion' in the application of synthetic chemicals ensued. Carson, however, remained unconvinced that pesticides underpinned the farm production required to sustain a burgeoning population (pages 6–7).[19] As a British agricultural researcher observed in 1998: 'Pesticides and inorganic fertilizers have got us into a situation where farming looks like a nineteenth century smokestack industry'.[20] And in tones reminiscent of Carson, Colin Tudge has recently criticized agricultural science and technology that has become divorced from the principles and traditions of sound husbandry.[21]

As she repeatedly emphasized in the storm that followed in the wake of her book, Carson did not call for a ban on chemical pesticides. She pleaded for a more informed and measured use of these substances. Her sensitivity for, and popularization of, 'the ecological web of life' encompassed a criticism of modern science and technology (pages 4–5). 'This is,' she observed, 'an era of specialists, each of whom sees his own problem and is unaware of or intolerant of the larger frame into which it fits. It is also an era dominated by industry, in which the right to make a dollar at whatever cost is seldom challenged.'[22] With this sentiment, Carson became the 'spiritual grandmother…to the whole counter-cultural rejection of technocracy' in the 1960s.[23] For her, this was part of a longer-running campaign to bridge the chasm between what C P Snow had called the 'two cultures' in his Rede lecture of 1959. By wedding her talents as a

---

[19] See Carson R. (1962; rept. 1987): 9.

[20] Simmons I G. (2001) *An Environmental History of Great Britain: From 10 000 years ago to present.* Edinburgh: Edinburgh University Press, 258–70.

[21] Tudge C. (2003) *So Shall we Reap.* London: Allen Lane.

[22] Carson R. (1962; rept. 1997): 13.

[23] See Marwick A. (1998) *The Sixties: Cultural Revolution in Britain, France, Italy, and the United States, c.1958–c.1974.* Oxford: Oxford University Press, 88. For an historical exploration of the relationship between insect control, professional ambitions and ecology, see Palladino P. (1996) *Entomology, Ecology and Agriculture: The making of scientific careers in North America, 1885–1985.* Amsterdam: Harwood Academic Publishers. For the British context, see Sheail J. (1985) *Pesticides and Nature Conservation: The British experience 1950–1975.* Oxford: Clarendon Press.

literary intellectual to her scientific knowledge, Carson aspired to replace an economic with an ecological approach to insecticides (pages 8–9).[24]

With the increasing emphasis on lifestyle choices and personal responsibility for health, it has become difficult to shift the focus from managing individual health to controlling the influences of the world around us in an ecologically informed manner (pages 21–22).[25] Rachel Carson embodied some of these tensions. Undoubtedly embarrassed by the cultural freight of some perceived personal failing, she never used the word 'cancer' or 'malignant' in relation to the disease from which she suffered in tragically ironic silence. But she referred directly to the threat of cancer from chemical insecticides in two of the chapters of *Silent Spring*, on which she was working at the time.[26] Eighteen months after the publication of *Silent Spring*, and 40 years ago this month [April 2004], Rachel Carson died from cancer. By raising our 'toxic consciousness', she contributed to a shift in perception of Western society. Whereas once defined by what it produced, Western culture is now defined by the waste and pollution that it generates. The Cold War era that gave birth to *Silent Spring* has been supplanted by 'the Age of the Environment'.[27]

John Clark
St Andrews

---

[24] Graham F Jr. (1970) *Since Silent Spring.* Greenwich: Fawcett Publications, 63.

[25] See Davis D. (2002) *When Smoke Ran Like Water: Tales of environmental deception and the battle against pollution.* Oxford: Perseus Press, xvi–xix.

[26] See Lear L. (1997): 368. In addition, see Sontag S. (1991) *Illness as Metaphor* and *AIDS and Its Metaphors.* London: Penguin Books.

[27] Deitering C. (1996) The Postnatural Novel: Toxic consciousness in the fiction of the 1980s, in Glotfelty C, Fromm H. (eds). *The Ecocriticism Reader: Landmarks in literary ecology.* Athens and London: University of Georgia Press, 196–203; Wilson E O. (2000) The Age of the Environment (suggestion for new name for post-Cold War era). *Foreign Policy*, Summer 2000.

ACKNOWLEDGEMENTS

We are particularly grateful to Dr Robert Flanagan, who assisted with the organization of the meeting, provided many of the names of individuals to be invited and helped decide on the topics to be discussed. We also thank Professor Tony Dayan for his excellent chairing of the occasion and for his help with the planning of the meeting. We are equally grateful to Dr John Clark for writing the introduction to these published proceedings. We thank Mr Richard Barnett for bibliographic research.

As with all our meetings, we depend a great deal on our colleagues at the Wellcome Trust to ensure their smooth running: the Audiovisual department, the Medical Photographic Library and Mrs Tracy Tillotson; Ms Julie Wood, who has supervised the design and production of this volume, our indexer, Ms Liza Furnival, our readers, Ms Lucy Moore, Mr Simon Reynolds and Mrs Lois Reynolds. We also thank Dr Robert Flanagan who read through an earlier draft of the transcript. Mrs Jaqui Carter is our transcriber, and Mrs Wendy Kutner and Mrs Lois Reynolds assist us in running the meetings. Finally we thank the Wellcome Trust for supporting this programme.

Tilli Tansey

Daphne Christie

Wellcome Trust Centre for the History of Medicine at UCL

WITNESS SEMINARS:
MEETINGS AND PUBLICATIONS[1]

In 1990 the Wellcome Trust created a History of Twentieth Century Medicine Group, as part of the Academic Unit of the Wellcome Institute for the History of Medicine, to bring together clinicians, scientists, historians and others interested in contemporary medical history. Among a number of other initiatives the format of Witness Seminars, used by the Institute of Contemporary British History to address issues of recent political history, was adopted, to promote interaction between these different groups, to emphasize the potential of working jointly, and to encourage the creation and deposit of archival sources for present and future use. In June 1999 the Governors of the Wellcome Trust decided that it would be appropriate for the Academic Unit to enjoy a more formal academic affiliation and turned the Unit into the Wellcome Trust Centre for the History of Medicine at University College London from 1 October 2000. The Wellcome Trust continues to fund the Witness Seminar programme via its support for the Centre.

The Witness Seminar is a particularly specialized form of oral history, where several people associated with a particular set of circumstances or events are invited to come together to discuss, debate, and agree or disagree about their memories. To date, the History of Twentieth Century Medicine Group has held over 30 such meetings, most of which have been published, as listed on pages xv–xxi.

Subjects are usually proposed by, or through, members of the Programme Committee of the Group, and once an appropriate topic has been agreed, suitable participants are identified and invited. These inevitably lead to further contacts, and more suggestions of people to invite. As the organization of the meeting progresses, a flexible outline plan for the meeting is devised, usually with assistance from the meeting's chairman, and some participants are invited to 'set the ball rolling' on particular themes, by speaking for a short period to initiate and stimulate further discussion.

Each meeting is fully recorded, the tapes are transcribed and the unedited transcript is immediately sent to every participant. Each is asked to check his or

---

[1] The following text also appears in the 'Introduction' to recent volumes of *Wellcome Witnesses to Twentieth Century Medicine* published by the Wellcome Trust and the Wellcome Trust Centre for the History of Medicine at University College London.

her own contributions and to provide brief biographical details. The editors turn the transcript into readable text, and participants' minor corrections and comments are incorporated into that text, while biographical and bibliographical details are added as footnotes, as are more substantial comments and additional material provided by participants. The final scripts are then sent to every contributor, accompanied by forms assigning copyright to the Wellcome Trust. Copies of all additional correspondence received during the editorial process are deposited with the records of each meeting in Archives and Manuscripts, Wellcome Library, London.

As with all our meetings, we hope that even if the precise details of some of the technical sections are not clear to the nonspecialist, the sense and significance of the events are understandable. Our aim is for the volumes that emerge from these meetings to inform those with a general interest in the history of modern medicine and medical science; to provide historians with new insights, fresh material for study, and further themes for research; and to emphasize to the participants that events of the recent past, of their own working lives, are of proper and necessary concern to historians.

HISTORY OF TWENTIETH CENTURY MEDICINE WITNESS SEMINARS, 1993–2004

1993   **Monoclonal antibodies**
Organizers: Dr E M Tansey and Dr Peter Catterall

1994   **The early history of renal transplantation**
Organizer: Dr Stephen Lock

Pneumoconiosis of coal workers
Organizer: Dr E M Tansey

1995   **Self and non-self: A history of autoimmunity**
Organizers: Sir Christopher Booth and Dr E M Tansey

Ashes to ashes: The history of smoking and health
Organizers: Dr Stephen Lock and Dr E M Tansey

Oral contraceptives
Organizers: Dr Lara Marks and Dr E M Tansey

Endogenous opiates
Organizer: Dr E M Tansey

1996   **Committee on Safety of Drugs**
Organizers: Dr Stephen Lock and Dr E M Tansey

Making the body more transparent: The impact of nuclear magnetic resonance and magnetic resonance imaging
Organizer: Sir Christopher Booth

1997   **Research in General Practice**
Organizers: Dr Ian Tait and Dr E M Tansey

Drugs in psychiatric practice
Organizers: Dr David Healy and Dr E M Tansey

The MRC Common Cold Unit
Organizers: Dr David Tyrrell and Dr E M Tansey

The first heart transplant in the UK
Organizer: Professor Tom Treasure

1998	**Haemophilia: Recent history of clinical management** Organizers: Professor Christine Lee and Dr E M Tansey
	Obstetric ultrasound: Historical perspectives Organizers: Dr Malcolm Nicolson, Mr John Fleming and Dr E M Tansey
	Post penicillin antibiotics Organizers: Dr Robert Bud and Dr E M Tansey
	Clinical research in Britain, 1950–1980 Organizers: Dr David Gordon and Dr E M Tansey
1999	**Intestinal absorption** Organizers: Sir Christopher Booth and Dr E M Tansey
	The MRC Epidemiology Unit (South Wales) Organizers: Dr Andy Ness and Dr E M Tansey
	Neonatal intensive care Organizers: Professor Osmund Reynolds and Dr E M Tansey
	British contributions to medicine in Africa after the Second World War Organizers: Dr Mary Dobson, Dr Maureen Malowany, Dr Gordon Cook and Dr E M Tansey
2000	**Childhood asthma, and beyond** Organizers: Dr Chris O'Callaghan and Dr Daphne Christie
	Peptic ulcer: Rise and fall Organizers: Sir Christopher Booth, Professor Roy Pounder and Dr E M Tansey
	Maternal care Organizers: Dr Irvine Loudon and Dr Daphne Christie
2001	**Leukaemia** Organizers: Professor Sir David Weatherall, Professor John Goldman, Sir Christopher Booth and Dr Daphne Christie
	The MRC Applied Psychology Unit Organizers: Dr Geoff Bunn and Dr Daphne Christie
	Genetic testing Organizers: Professor Doris Zallen and Dr Daphne Christie

Foot and mouth disease: the 1967 outbreak and its aftermath
Organizers: Dr Abigail Woods, Dr Daphne Christie and
Dr David Aickin

2002   Environmental toxicology: The legacy of *Silent Spring*
Organizers: Dr Robert Flanagan and Dr Daphne Christie

Cystic fibrosis
Organizers: Dr James Littlewood and Dr Daphne Christie

Innovation in pain management
Organizers: Professor David Clark and Dr Daphne Christie

2003   Thrombolysis
Organizers: Mr Robert Arnott and Dr Daphne Christie

Beyond the asylum: Anti-psychiatry and care in the community
Organizers: Dr Mark Jackson and Dr Daphne Christie

The Rhesus factor and disease prevention
Organizers: Professor Doris Zallen and Dr Daphne Christie

Platelets in thrombosis and other disorders
Organizers: Professor Gustav Born and Dr Daphne Christie

2004   Short course chemotherapy for tuberculosis
Organizers: Dr Owen McCarthy and Dr Daphne Christie

Prenatal corticosteroids for reducing morbidity and mortality
associated with preterm birth
Organizers: Sir Iain Chalmers and Dr Daphne Christie

PUBLISHED MEETINGS

"…Few books are so intellectually stimulating or uplifting".
Journal of the Royal Society of Medicine (1999) **92:** 206–8,
review of vols 1 and 2

*"…This is oral history at its best…all the volumes make compulsive
reading…they are, primarily, important historical records".*
British Medical Journal (2002) **325:** 1119, review of the series

Technology transfer in Britain: The case of monoclonal antibodies
Self and non-self: A history of autoimmunity
Endogenous opiates
The Committee on Safety of Drugs
In: Tansey E M, Catterall P P, Christie D A, Willhoft S V, Reynolds L A. (eds)
(1997) *Wellcome Witnesses to Twentieth Century Medicine.* Volume 1. London:
The Wellcome Trust, 135pp. ISBN 1 869835 79 4

Making the human body transparent: The impact of NMR and MRI
Research in General Practice
Drugs in psychiatric practice
The MRC Common Cold Unit
In: Tansey E M, Christie D A, Reynolds L A. (eds) (1998) *Wellcome Witnesses
to Twentieth Century Medicine.* Volume 2. London: The Wellcome Trust,
282pp. ISBN 1 869835 39 5

Early heart transplant surgery in the UK
In: Tansey E M, Reynolds L A. (eds) (1999) *Wellcome Witnesses to Twentieth
Century Medicine.* Volume 3. London: The Wellcome Trust, 72pp.
ISBN 1 841290 07 6

Haemophilia: Recent history of clinical management
In: Tansey E M, Christie D A. (eds) (1999) *Wellcome Witnesses to Twentieth Century
Medicine.* Volume 4. London: The Wellcome Trust, 90pp. ISBN 1 841290 08 4

Looking at the unborn: Historical aspects of obstetric ultrasound
In: Tansey E M, Christie D A. (eds) (2000) *Wellcome Witnesses to Twentieth Century
Medicine.* Volume 5. London: The Wellcome Trust, 80pp. ISBN 1 841290 11 4

Post penicillin antibiotics: From acceptance to resistance?

In: Tansey E M, Reynolds L A. (eds) (2000) *Wellcome Witnesses to Twentieth Century Medicine*. Volume 6. London: The Wellcome Trust, 71pp. ISBN 1 841290 12 2

Clinical research in Britain, 1950–1980

In: Reynolds L A, Tansey E M. (eds) (2000) *Wellcome Witnesses to Twentieth Century Medicine*. Volume 7. London: The Wellcome Trust, 74pp. ISBN 1 841290 16 5

Intestinal absorption

In: Christie D A, Tansey E M. (eds) (2000) *Wellcome Witnesses to Twentieth Century Medicine*. Volume 8. London: The Wellcome Trust, 81pp. ISBN 1 841290 17 3

Neonatal intensive care

In: Christie D A, Tansey E M. (eds) (2001) *Wellcome Witnesses to Twentieth Century Medicine*. Volume 9. London: The Wellcome Trust Centre for the History of Medicine at UCL, 84pp. ISBN 0 854840 76 1

British contributions to medical research and education in Africa after the Second World War

In: Reynolds L A, Tansey E M. (eds) (2001) *Wellcome Witnesses to Twentieth Century Medicine*. Volume 10. London: The Wellcome Trust Centre for the History of Medicine at UCL, 93pp. ISBN 0 854840 77 X

Childhood asthma and beyond

In: Reynolds L A, Tansey E M. (eds) (2001) *Wellcome Witnesses to Twentieth Century Medicine*. Volume 11. London: The Wellcome Trust Centre for the History of Medicine at UCL, 74pp. ISBN 0 854840 78 8

Maternal care

In: Christie D A, Tansey E M. (eds) (2001) *Wellcome Witnesses to Twentieth Century Medicine*. Volume 12. London: The Wellcome Trust Centre for the History of Medicine at UCL, 88pp. ISBN 0 854840 79 6

Population-based research in south Wales: The MRC Pneumoconiosis Research Unit and the MRC Epidemiology Unit

In: Ness A R, Reynolds L A, Tansey E M. (eds) (2002) *Wellcome Witnesses to Twentieth Century Medicine*. Volume 13. London: The Wellcome Trust Centre for the History of Medicine at UCL, 74pp. ISBN 0 854840 81 8

Peptic ulcer: Rise and fall
In: Christie D A, Tansey E M. (eds) (2002) *Wellcome Witnesses to Twentieth Century Medicine.* Volume 14. London: The Wellcome Trust Centre for the History of Medicine at UCL, 143pp. ISBN 0 854840 84 2

Leukaemia
In: Christie D A, Tansey E M. (eds) (2003) *Wellcome Witnesses to Twentieth Century Medicine.* Volume 15. London: The Wellcome Trust Centre for the History of Medicine at UCL, 86pp. ISBN 0 85484 087 7

The MRC Applied Psychology Unit
In: Reynolds L A, Tansey E M. (eds) (2003) *Wellcome Witnesses to Twentieth Century Medicine.* Volume 16. London: The Wellcome Trust Centre for the History of Medicine at UCL, 94pp. ISBN 0 85484 088 5

Genetic testing
In: Christie D A, Tansey E M. (eds) (2003) *Wellcome Witnesses to Twentieth Century Medicine.* Volume 17. London: The Wellcome Trust Centre for the History of Medicine at UCL, 130pp. ISBN 0 85484 094 X

Foot and mouth disease: The 1967 outbreak and its aftermath
In: Reynolds L A, Tansey E M. (eds) (2003) *Wellcome Witnesses to Twentieth Century Medicine.* Volume 18. London: The Wellcome Trust Centre for the History of Medicine at UCL, 114pp. ISBN 0 85484 096 6

Environmental toxicology: The legacy of *Silent Spring*
In: Christie D A, Tansey E M. (eds) (2004) *Wellcome Witnesses to Twentieth Century Medicine.* Volume 19. London: The Wellcome Trust Centre for the History of Medicine at UCL, this volume. ISBN 0 85484 091 5

Cystic fibrosis
In: Christie D A, Tansey E M. (eds) (2004) *Wellcome Witnesses to Twentieth Century Medicine.* Volume 20. London: The Wellcome Trust Centre for the History of Medicine at UCL, 120pp. ISBN 0 85484 086 9

Innovation in pain management
In: Reynolds L A, Tansey E M. (eds) (2004) *Wellcome Witnesses to Twentieth Century Medicine.* Volume 21. London: The Wellcome Trust Centre for the History of Medicine at UCL, in press. ISBN 0 85484 097 4

The Rhesus factor and disease prevention

In: Zallen D, Christie D A, Tansey E M. (eds) (2004) *Wellcome Witnesses to Twentieth Century Medicine.* Volume 22. London: The Wellcome Trust Centre for the History of Medicine at UCL, in press. ISBN 0 85484 099 0

Platelets in thrombosis and other disorders

In: Reynolds L A, Tansey E M. (eds) (2005) *Wellcome Witnesses to Twentieth Century Medicine.* Volume 23. London: The Wellcome Trust Centre for the History of Medicine at UCL, in press.

Short course chemotherapy for tuberculosis

In: Christie D A, Tansey E M. (eds) (2005) *Wellcome Witnesses to Twentieth Century Medicine.* Volume 24. London: The Wellcome Trust Centre for the History of Medicine at UCL, in press.

Volumes 1–12 cost £5.00 plus postage, with volumes 13–20 at £10 each. Orders of four or more volumes receive a 20 per cent discount. All 20 published volumes in the series are available at the special price of £115 plus postage. To order a copy contact t.tillotson@wellcome.ac.uk or by phone: +44 (0)20 7611 8486; or fax: +44 (0)20 7611 8703.

Other publications

Technology transfer in Britain: The case of monoclonal antibodies
In: Tansey E M, Catterall P P. (1993) *Contemporary Record* 9: 409–44.

Monoclonal antibodies: A witness seminar on contemporary medical history
In: Tansey E M, Catterall P P. (1994) *Medical History* 38: 322–7.

Chronic pulmonary disease in South Wales coalmines: An eye-witness account of the MRC surveys (1937–42)
In: P D'Arcy Hart, edited and annotated by E M Tansey. (1998) *Social History of Medicine* 11: 459–68.

Ashes to Ashes – The history of smoking and health
In: Lock S P, Reynolds L A, Tansey E M. (eds) (1998) Amsterdam: Rodopi BV, 228pp. ISBN 90420 0396 0 (Hfl 125) (hardback). Reprinted 2003.

Witnessing medical history. An interview with Dr Rosemary Biggs
Professor Christine Lee and Dr Charles Rizza (interviewers). (1998) *Haemophilia* 4: 769–77.

ENVIRONMENTAL TOXICOLOGY:
THE LEGACY OF *SILENT SPRING*

The transcript of a Witness Seminar held by the Wellcome Trust Centre for the History of Medicine at UCL, London, on 12 March 2002

Edited by D A Christie and E M Tansey

ENVIRONMENTAL TOXICOLOGY:
THE LEGACY OF *SILENT SPRING*

Participants

Professor Sir Colin Berry
Sir Christopher Booth
Professor Richard Carter
Dr Peter Corcoran
Professor Tony Dayan (Chair)
Professor Peter Farmer
Dr Robert Flanagan
Dr Peter Hunter

Mr Stanley Johnson
Professor James Lovelock
Professor Robert Maynard
Dr Ingar Palmlund
Dr Dennis Simms
Professor Robert Smith
Professor Frank Woods

Among those attending the meeting: Professor John Caldwell, Mrs Emma Eagles, Mr Stephen Lacey, Dr Joanna Reynolds, Ms Helen Smethurst, Mr Timothy Stentiford, Dr Janice Taverne

Apologies include: Sir Donald Acheson, Professor Ross Anderson, Professor Peter Blain, Professor Peter Brimblecombe, Miss Frances Cairncross, Professor Peter Calow, Professor David Coggon, Dr Mark Crane, Professor Donald Davies, Professor Paul Elliott, Dr John Fawell, Dr Robin Fielder, Professor Stephen Holgate, Professor Tim Jackson, Professor Martin Johnson, Dr Norman King, Professor Patrick Lawther, Professor Anthony McMichael, Dr David Morgan, Dr Angus Nicoll, Sir Jonathon Porritt, Dr Iain Purchase, Professor Lewis Smith

Professor Tony Dayan: Good afternoon, colleagues. I have a feeling I am here as, I think what the historians would call, the artefact, as I have been surrounded by the environment for a long while. The intention is to ask people to talk about the issues, the concerns, the problems and the actions, very much as they saw them at the time and clearly as they now recall them. We will lead on, I hope, to the present and the future, but taking very much of that message of the past. For convenience we have divided the afternoon into two parts: one predominantly concerned with pesticides and their immediate problems and effects; and in the latter half of the afternoon we will go on to more general areas related to air and water pollution.

These topics must be taken broadly. We are concerned with human health, the environment and environmental health, and the health of other living systems – ecology in the broadest fashion. I am looking forward to hearing what you are going to say. Let's start then with Professor Lovelock.

Professor James Lovelock: Thank you, Chairman. Rachel Carson's story[1] must go a long way back in time. I could find no classical references,[2] and I suppose environmental concern started in the eighteenth and nineteenth centuries, when the Industrial Revolution intensified agriculture and led to much greater food production. But, of course, there were also appalling events, among them the Irish famine, caused by potato blight.[3] It was these that led us to use chemical agents for pests and fungi control. In the nineteenth century these included substances like lead arsenate, nicotine and coal-tar dyes. Most of them were universally toxic, although a few were benign, like the Bordeaux mixture of

---

[1] See Carson (1962).

[2] Dr Dennis Simms wrote: 'The devastation wrought in classical times to fauna was on a large scale. When Hitler invaded Greece, there were no lions left to harass his supplies as they had done to Xerxes' troops. But, in addition to the destruction of flora and fauna, deforestation and soil erosion, there was environmental pollution from similar processes to those of the recent past. Many writers were aware of the resultant dangers: Vitruvius (*De Architectura*) described how to obtain clean water free from contaminants. Being sent to the silver mines at Laurion near Athens and the mercury mines in Iberia was recognized as a death sentence. Lucretius described the effects of gold mining on the miners. The remedies offered by the Greek poet, Nicander, for toxic metal poisoning were disgusting, dangerous and always futile. But although outbreaks of lead poisoning were common, there is no sound evidence that it caused the downfall of the Roman Empire.' E-mail to Mrs Lois Reynolds, 23 May 2003. See also Hughes (1994).

[3] In 1845 the Irish potato crop was devastated by an attack of 'late blight', now known to be the plant pathogen *Phytophthora infestans*; see Ristaino (2001). See also Kinealy (1997); Grada (1999).

sulphur and copper, which was effective against fungi.[4] Another almost benign agent was pyrethrin, which came along a bit later.[5]

Up until the Second World War the range of chemical weapons that could be used for pest control was almost as limited as the range of drugs that were available to cure infectious disease. I think it was Lewis Thomas who said that there were only three medicines before the mid-1930s that were any use at all.[6] Then in 1939 the Swiss chemist, Müller, discovered the potent insecticidal properties of DDT.[7] Interestingly, this was a compound first synthesized in the previous century, but no one had noticed its potential at that time. It was so powerful, yet apparently harmless to humans, that it was used on a grand scale towards the end of the Second World War and subsequently. It was used to kill lice, cut short epidemics of typhus and it proved to be a potent agent in malaria control. It was said to have saved more lives than any other chemical, and Müller was awarded the Nobel Prize for Physiology or Medicine in 1948, I think most people at the time thought most deservedly.[8]

The 1940s and 1950s were, of course, times of innocence. We all believed that science was benign and that eventually the sensible use of chemicals would set humankind free from pests and disease. But it was also, of course, a time when many new herbicides and pesticides were invented, including the organophosphates.[9] The

---

[4] Professor James Lovelock wrote: 'The original Bordeaux mixture was discovered accidentally in 1882; it was made from calcium hydroxide, copper sulphate and water. It is still used as a fungicidal wash or spray to treat orchard trees (source *Encyclopaedia Britannica* 2002).' Letter to Dr Daphne Christie, 9 December 2003.

[5] Pyrethrum, an extract of the chrysanthemum and otherwise known as Persian Insect Powder, was used as an insecticide from the early nineteenth century. Pyrethrin insecticides came on to the market in the late 1960s and early 1970s. See McLaughlin (1973) and page 96.

[6] Quinine (malaria), emetine (amoebic dysentery), thymol (intestinal hookworm) and arsphenamine (syphilis). See Thomas L. (1983): 13; Russell (2001). See also correspondence from Dr Peter Hunter to Dr Daphne Christie, 30 March 2004.

[7] DDT [1,1-bis(4-chlorophenyl)-2,2,2-trichloroethane] was first synthesized by Othmar Zeidler in 1874. It was first used on a large scale by the US Army in Italy in 1943, and after the Second World War was taken up across the world as part of the Eighth World Health Assembly's global Malaria Eradication Program. By 1962 over 80 million kilograms of DDT were used each year. By 1970 DDT was being supplanted by more quickly degraded, less toxic agents. Its use was banned in a number of countries., in the USA from 1972 and from 1986 in the UK. See Dunlap (1981); Jackson (1998); Tren and Bate (2001).

[8] Paul Müller received the 1948 Nobel Prize for 'his discovery of the high efficiency of DDT as a contact poison against several arthropods'. See Müller, (1948, 1955); Quiroga (1990): 416–19.

[9] The first organophosphate pesticides were developed during the Second World War at I G Farben's chemical plant at Auschwitz. Malathion came on to the market in 1950. See Najera *et al.* (1967).

illusion broke in 1962 when Rachel Carson published her seminal book *Silent Spring.*[10] Like all her books, it was beautifully written and it became a bestseller, but the message was apocalyptic: if we went on using chemical pesticides bird life would soon become extinct.

Well, I played a minor, possibly significant, part in this story. I had invented in 1956 at the National Institute for Medical Research at Mill Hill a device called the electron capture detector (ECD).[11] It was exquisitely but selectively sensitive to unpleasant substances, including halogenated compounds, and it could detect them directly in biological materials with minimal prior sample preparation. By 1960 it was available from scientific instrument manufacturers in Europe and the USA, and was widely used. Strangely, there's no mention of this device in Rachel Carson's book. She mentions only wet chemical methods,[12] whose accuracy would have been in doubt particularly at the parts per million levels she was talking about. It seems probable that the chemists who advised her on the results of pesticide analysis were aware of the ECD, but stuck with their familiar methods, which to them seemed the sensible thing to do.

It was not long before the electron capture detector became the standard method for pesticide and herbicide analysis. Its disadvantage was that it was much too sensitive. As little as a few hundred thousand molecules of a pesticide like dieldrin[13] or DDT can be detected, or in other words a few

---

[10] Carson (1962).

[11] The electron capture device (ECD) is the most sensitive gas chromatographic detector for halogen-containing compounds such as chlorofluorocarbons (CFCs). Lovelock's first model of the device was made from scrap materials and a spark-plug. Lovelock's account of his early career and the invention of the ECD can be found at resurgence.gn.apc.org/issues/lovelock187.htm (site accessed 12 September 2003). See also Lovelock (1997).

[12] 'Wet chemical methods' were used in air-quality monitoring prior to the mid-1960s. Ambient air was drawn through a reagent solution, removing a particular pollutant via chemical reaction with the reagent. Quantitative UV analysis was then carried out in the laboratory. These methods had a number of limitations, including poor temporal resolution due to the long sampling times required to achieve the necessary sensitivity, and poor selectivity due to interference from other pollutants in the air samples.

[13] Dieldrin is one of a group of organophosphate pesticides which are structurally related to DDT. From the 1950s until the 1970s dieldrin was widely used as a pesticide in the USA and western Europe. However, like DDT, dieldrin was found to accumulate in food chains and has been linked to chronic disease in humans. In 1974 the US Environmental Protection Agency banned all uses of dieldrin except for termite control, and it was banned completely in 1987. See, for example, Carson (1962): 93–95, 130, 154, 175.

femtograms.[14] At this sensitivity pesticides can be found in natural vegetation, even from a remote area such as the islands off Antarctica. As soon as a quantity is attached to a measurement, sadly it seems to acquire a spurious significance. Numeracy is unfortunately not common and when it is said that pesticides have been found in a foodstuff, the unwise immediately assume that it's unhealthy to eat, regardless of the fact that the quantity may be quite infinitesimal. It is interesting to me that the same people often also believe in the curative powers of homeopathic medicine. The politicians didn't help, because some of them demanded 'zero' levels for toxic agents. When you can measure femtograms, 'zero' becomes extremely small. We were carried away by the promise of science in the first half of the last century, but I think we have gone much too far in the second half in denigrating it.

Dayan: Thank you. You have raised many issues for us to talk about. Sir Colin Berry has promised to lead us off on some aspects of pesticides.

Professor Sir Colin Berry: One of the important things I think we have forgotten in much of the debate that has ended up by vilifying chemicals, is that between 1850 and 1900 around 200 million hectares of grassland were converted into grain fields in the USA alone, and there was a comparable change in Russia and Australia, and some of the South American countries.[15] This change in land use and the use of agriculture machinery increasing world population. But nobody's making any more land, or at least if you do (as in Holland or in Singapore) it's far too expensive to use for farming. So we needed another set of advances to go on feeding people.

Those of you who have seen Vaclav Smil's book on the nitrogen-fixing process[16] will know that he wrote that if we were to provide the average 1995 per capita food supply using the 1900 level of agricultural productivity, we could only feed 2.4 billion people, or about 40 per cent of those alive today. Without considering pesticides or genetic engineering, there is a very good illustration of how simple farming techniques and the use of land have changed. Indeed the pressure nowadays is to return more land to wilderness rather than to increase the use of land. The apocalyptic view that was taken in Rachel Carson's book was matched

---

[14] A femtogram is 10^{-15} g. See also note 50.

[15] Smil (2001): ch. 8.

[16] Smil (2001).

by another one on the food issue by Professor Paul Ehrlich who, in 1971 in *The Population Bomb* wrote:

> The battle to feed all of humanity is over. The famines of the 1970s are upon us – and hundreds of millions of more people are going to starve to death before this decade is out.[17]

This shows the value of nonsense. *The Population Bomb* sold very well: 3 million copies. Apocalyptic warnings are very much in favour with those who are anxious about things.

So the changes involved in the way in which farming is practised now have included selective breeding of crops, the use of artificial nitrogen and importantly, I think, the prevention of pest-related crop failure and losses. Losses due to food spoilage, and the prevention of the formation of toxins in food as a consequence of both pests and spoilage, including losses in transport and storage, have been reduced enormously by chemical treatment. But, as has already been pointed out, it is the chemicals, rather than the microbiological agents and their problems that the chemicals are designed to eliminate, that have attracted opprobrium. I think it will be worth exploring how it is that we got to this situation, bearing in mind the enormous benefits we gain from modern agriculture.

As a comparison, if you slash and burn the forest in the Amazon and then move on, having grown crops, you can support about one person per hectare with a 25-year recovery cycle. In southern China, before the Second World War, intensive agriculture, by which I mean the use of human and animal excreta, of cyanobacterial fixation of nitrogen in carp ponds, with the dead and rotting material from those ponds put on the land and so on, supported about ten people per hectare with a huge human disease burden imposed on the population by using that kind of agricultural methodology.[18] And yet modern agriculture supports 45 people per hectare every year,[19] and although there are undoubtedly adverse consequences, that's a sobering comparison.

Dayan: Dr Corcoran, you had a long involvement with the control of toxic chemicals and we have to regard even pesticides selective for particular properties as they are, as being toxic.

---

[17] See Ehrlich (1971): ix.

[18] See Zhu *et al.* (1997): 328.

[19] Smil (2001): ch. 8.

Dr Peter Corcoran: My role on the Advisory Committee on Pesticides (ACP) was as a departmental assessor.[20] Assessors represent Ministers, who are finally responsible for agreeing whether a pesticide can be used or not. So assessors have to balance the purely scientific views represented by the excellent members of the committee, including of course yourself, Chairman, with what they judge will be the political view. In my experience the approvals procedures for pesticides came to scientifically valid conclusions that were also politically acceptable at the time. By and large the recommendations of the ACP were accepted both by Ministers and by the public,[21] apart from a relatively small number of people who were simply opposed to pesticides and eat organically. So I would say that science did feed into the decision-making process, and I am sure that the overall decisions that were reached were sensible ones.

Dayan: One of the things that strikes me, listening particularly to the first three speakers, knowing what little I do of that era, is that many of us became, at least initially, very concerned about human health and its protection (with the exception of Rachel Carson) unless I am showing my own particular bias. There was rather less concern with ecological health and of the non-human living systems. Now I don't know whether I am wrong there, or whether there was as much concern with these other systems, despite Dr Carson's very strident call. How did that come about?

Lovelock: My memory is that you are completely right. There was very little concern about world ecology before Rachel Carson's book.[22] We were all in a humanist frame of mind and the good of mankind seemed to be a sufficient aim for us to work towards. Certainly in the Medical Research Council [MRC] I don't think anybody seemed to feel that what they were doing could even conceivably be thought of as harmful to the environment.

Berry: I agree, I think that was true. I think that it was because we had this humanocentric view of things. The success of DDT at the end of the Second World War in breaking up the typhus outbreak which was devastating southern

---

[20] The Advisory Committee on Pesticides (ACP) was established in 1985 under section 16(7) of the 1985 Food and Environmental Protection Act. It advises the British government on pesticide regulation in the UK.

[21] Advisory Committee on Pesticides (2002).

[22] See Whorton (1974) for a discussion of the pre-*Silent Spring* ecology movement. See also Gunter and Harris (1998).

Europe[23] and the enormous advances in malaria prevention in Ceylon, when it looked as if it would become a malaria-free island,[24] were seen as very real advances. Those successes distracted people, despite what we have said about the sense of loss of magical process in science. Max Weber,[25] a sociologist, wrote of the loss of 'entzauberung',[26] and he certainly thought that people were giving up on science. It wasn't just that attitude, it was, I think, simply that nobody had thought about adverse effects because so much benefit was coming in a way that was easily observable.

Mr Stanley Johnson: I was involved at a very early date in the European Union's (EU) environmental programme – then it was the European Economic Community (EEC), it's got rather grander recently.[27] Its first environmental programme was drawn up at the beginning of 1973, shortly after the enlargement of the EEC from the then six members to nine members. The UK joined on 1 January 1973,[28] and I do recall that one of the issues facing us as we drew up the first environmental action programme was how to deal with the question of environmental toxicity. I think I would be right to say that at least in the first and second environmental action programmes, 1973–76 and 1976–80, the emphasis was very much on the impact of toxic chemicals, including pesticides, on human health.

Why do I say that? Partly because the EEC was drawing on the existing set of criteria. When I use the word 'criteria' I am using it in the rather special sense that the EU's first environmental action programme used it, that is to say, an effort to describe a dose–effect relationship. The idea was that at a certain level

---

[23] See Russell (1999) for the politics of DDT use during the Second World War.

[24] See Jackson (1998); Packard (1998) for the global Malaria Eradication Program in the 1950s.

[25] Max Weber (1864–1920) argued for a scientific and value-free approach to research, yet highlighted the importance of meaning and consciousness in understanding social action. See Parsons (1976); Turner (1992).

[26] Disenchantment; a word commonly used by nineteenth-century German intellectuals to describe the perception of an emotional or spiritual void in modern society. See Boyer (2001).

[27] Mr Stanley Johnson wrote: 'The Treaty of Maastricht (1992) introduced new forms of cooperation between the member-state governments – for example on defence, and in the area of "justice and home affairs". By adding this intergovernmental cooperation to the existing "community" system, the Maastricht Treaty created the European Union (EU).' Note on draft transcript, 12 December 2003.

[28] The UK entered the EEC during Edward Heath's Conservative government in 1973, along with Denmark and Ireland.

the presence of a particular chemical in the environment would be harmful to human health. I stress human health. In that first programme we picked a number of chemicals, obviously the more obvious ones, but some slightly less obvious, like vanadium.[29] Now in moving on this field of activity, we were very much inspired by the work which the WHO [World Health Organization] had done in the 1960s in drawing up its criteria documents, including, of course, standards on air pollution and certain water pollutants.[30]

Within its first few years the EU defined dose–effect relationships for the presence of chemicals in the environment, and it did so having in mind human health. It's only been, I would say, in the last ten or 15 years – but Peter Corcoran and Dennis Simms will be able to correct me on this – that the EU has made a wider effort to try to define environmental standards based also on the effect of pollutants on the environment as a whole, including, of course, the aquatic and terrestrial environments, and this has been a much more complicated exercise.

It has been a two-fold approach. There's been an attempt to define environmental quality standards, which, as I have said, tended to be largely health quality standards, but at the same time there was an attempt to define product standards. That gave rise to a whole array of environmental legislation emanating from the EU in the 1970s and 1980s to do with the presence of toxic, or potentially toxic, chemicals in products. Whether these were new chemical products, in which case there were EU procedures for the testing of these products, or whether they were existing chemical products, in which case whole procedures were laid down for the inventory and assessment of those products. So it became very, very complex altogether and, of course, the effort had always been to relate these product standards to the toxic burden in the environment as a whole.

The EU has never, I think, managed to solve the question of the use of animal testing as a proxy for defining danger to man. It has become a terrifically controversial issue and remains so today, and I would say it's one of the great challenges for legislators throughout the West to define systems of assessing toxicity that do not rely on animal tests.

---

[29] The environmental impact of vanadium, a toxic metal, remains poorly understood. It is present in a variety of compounds, most notably crude oil and petroleum, and high environmental levels of the element have been detected since the 1960s. However, some studies have suggested that vanadium is also an essential nutrient for certain groups of organisms. See, for example, Zaporowska and Wasilewski (1992); Nriagu (1998).

[30] See, for example, World Health Organization (1972).

Corcoran: May I expand a little and comment on some of the issues raised by others. When looking at the assessment of the impact of pesticides on human health and the environment, there is a fundamental difference between the acceptable risks to people and to the environment. The acceptable risk to consumers from pesticide residues, or to people using pesticides, is effectively zero, disregarding, for the moment, accidents. That's not so in the case of the environment; it is accepted in making an approval [by a safety committee] that a pesticide is going to have an impact on the environment.

In fact that's its whole purpose, that's exactly what it is supposed to do, and that impact is only part of the impact of intensive farming in general. The whole point of intensive farming is to change the environment, to grow food. So when looking at the environmental impact of pesticides, you have to balance the benefits and the known environmental factors, and to try to identify primary effects that are acceptable because they aim to improve agriculture, and the unintended secondary effects. So there is a fundamental difference between zero risk for human health and an acceptable risk for the environment.

Berry: I very much agree with what Peter says. I think we have another major failing that wasn't apparent to us in the past, and that is that we have tended to assume that there will be global solutions, which I am sure is wrong. If I can leap forward 40 years we now would begin to think very hard about using certain drugs in individuals when we know a good deal about their genetic make-up. There will be some people who can tolerate particular drugs that will kill others (a good example might have been Opren[31]). Now if it is possible to distinguish between which people it would kill and which it would aid, perhaps that means you use the drug differently. In the same way, the DDT decision that was made probably on (at least) suspicious data about American birds of prey,[32] had an enormous impact in other parts of the world and I think some of these ideas of zero risk in one society might be quite different in another society. We have been rather too imperialistic about some of our attitudes. That's something that may be an important historical change: we get better at deciding which is the risk–benefit

---

[31] Opren (benoxaprofen) is a non-steroidal anti-inflammatory drug (NSAID) used to treat arthritis, which has been shown to cause death from intestinal bleeding in some patients. See Anon. (1983).

[32] The idea that DDT was responsible for the declining population of many bird species because it thinned and weakened their eggshells was a central tenet of *Silent Spring*. This hypothesis was based on the work of Dr James DeWitt, who claimed that the eggs of quail and pheasants, which had been exposed to DDT over a long period, were much less likely to hatch. See DeWitt (1955, 1956).

analysis we are going to consider. I have just been reading something about the Botswana government's policy in tsetse-fly control and one of the telling statements in the documents is, 'What would happen to Botswana's tourist industry if one tourist died of sleeping sickness?'[33] It's a quite different perspective, organochlorine versus pyrethroid,[34] which we might adopt in Europe.

Professor Frank Woods: I wonder, Mr Chairman, if I might return to something that the first speaker said and is a very fundamental point: that when these effective chemicals were first introduced, there seemed to be a complete lack of interest in their environmental impact.[35] I am not surprised at that, because if you look at the whole history, particularly the history of European man's attitude towards the natural world – and I think it is very well summed up in Keith Thomas' book[36] – you will see that for many hundreds of years we have had a very materialistic view of the environment, that it was there for our benefit rather than the more recent, and, of course, more excellent view, that we are going to have to look after it. I am afraid that the environment has taken a chemical battering for at least 200 years and we have completely ignored it, because we had this view that it was there for our benefit.

Dayan: Do you feel that our attitude to the environment has been one of not just indifference, deliberate ignorance or unawareness perhaps until very recently, or is it that we knew there might be effects, and we didn't bother, because the direct human benefits were so clear that there was no need to worry about anything else?

Lovelock: To return, Chairman, to what you said earlier on, why did we have this change of heart? Since this seminar is about the history of the story, I think we shouldn't leave out of the account the other things that happened in relatively recent years, like the concern about the ozone layer and more recently about growing greenhouse gas accumulation.[37] These, I think, made people for the first time aware that they were dealing with a global problem, and it fed back to Rachel

---

[33] From the first appearance of sleeping sickness in Botswana in 1934, outbreaks increased up to 1971. In 1973 aerial spraying with endosulfan coincided with a decline in the disease and in 1979 aerial spraying was shown to be effective in eliminating a threatened epidemic of sleeping sickness. See Davies (1982).

[34] In other words, the highly effective but extremely toxic and persistent organochlorine pesticides as opposed to the less effective but 'greener' pyrethroids.

[35] See page 8.

[36] Thomas K. (1983).

[37] Watson (2001).

Carson's story in a way that amplified it much faster than it otherwise would have been and brought it into the public consciousness right around the world. We are now much more aware that we are part of a small planet with limited resources.

Dayan: How much of that change in attitude has come from changes and improvement in basic scientific understanding? You can't investigate a problem until first of all you recognize that there is something, even if it's not well defined until you have some methods with which to explore it. I wondered if, say, going back to the 1960s, to Rachel Carson, her examples, particularly of birds, were ones that stood out very clearly for particular reasons. Perhaps ornithologists have been more quantitative than many other natural scientists for various reasons. How much do we just lack that basic understanding of the processes?

Professor Richard Carter: I think it's primarily a lack of understanding. It's interesting that Rachel Carson placed so much emphasis on birds: could she have made an equally attractive case with, shall we say, insects? I doubt that she would have made the general impact that she did. She chose a very good example.

Could I make a very brief comment about Keith Thomas' book, *Man and the Natural World*,[38] which was mentioned just now? In it he discusses variations between different approaches to the natural world – historical, social, religious, literary – and also different approaches in different countries in Europe. But he says very little about events after the 1800s.[39]

Dayan: Only perhaps in explaining some of the attitudes that we have. But I agree that it is not a direct analysis.

Dr Ingar Palmlund: My history goes back to the 1970s as well. I was Director of the Swedish Council of Environmental Information, and was working for the Swedish government in the no-man's land between science and politics at the time, developing computer support for governmental agencies and so forth.

I have two comments I would like to make. First, Rachel Carson's book is interesting in a way that we forgot for several decades; her book inspired a great deal of concern over cancer risks, carcinogenic compounds, but in fact most of her book deals with reproductive hazards. It wasn't until about seven or eight

---

[38] Thomas K. (1983).

[39] Dr Dennis Simms wrote: 'The book by Keith Thomas rarely goes beyond the mid-eighteenth century. The superstitions do, but he does not recognize this.' Letter to Dr Daphne Christie, 30 November 2003.

years ago when concerns over hormones in the environment, the endocrine disturbances that industrial chemicals might cause, that the interest in her book emerged again.[40] So in a way in our culture we selected the cancer hazard as a kind of a profile for funding, a basis for channelling money to research. That had a considerable impact on the developments.

The second point that I would like to make is that I believe that the United Nations Conference on the Environment in 1972 in Stockholm really was a landmark in raising awareness about the vulnerability of the planet and of environmental conditions.[41] The report that came from studies in southern Norway and Sweden of dying lakes inspired a great deal of concern.[42] After that UN conference, government politicians from all parts of the world went home to their countries and started developing legislation to control environmental problems, investing money in research and setting up agencies whose sole concern was the protection of the environment. I think that conference in a way has sustained the interest and the research in this area.

Dayan: Do you feel, though, that the wish to protect, and the legislative and regulatory means to protect, have actually marched to the same tune as the science? One would hope, one would expect that the science should be in advance, because you can't control what you don't know you want to control, and you don't know how to do so. I fear there may have been a basic mismatch there.

Palmlund: I think it's different in different areas. I have been fascinated to follow the politics of the global climate change debate. I should perhaps mention that I have been teaching international environment development politics at Tufts University in Boston, USA, recently. The world-view that climatologists have had for a long time brought them together at annual or even quarterly meetings which have made them share data across political frontiers in a way that many other scientists have not been able to communicate and compare their world-views and their understanding of what

---

[40] Carson (1962): 207–9.

[41] The United Nations Conference on the Human Environment took place in Stockholm from 5–16 June 1972, and produced a set of principles in the Stockholm Declaration that led to the founding of the United Nations Environment Programme. See www.unep.org/documents/default.asp?documentID=97 for the full text of the conference report (site accessed 25 September 2003). See also note 116.

[42] See, for example, *Green Issues*, a publication from the Norwegian Pollution Control Authority, www.rst2.edu/ties/acidrain/PDF/3effects/ef9.pdf (site accessed 5 December 2003).

was happening.[43] I think that has had an impact on the political developments. The climatologists, after scientific meetings in the 1970s, went back to their home governments and took it as their responsibility to instruct politicians about what they understood about global climate change. I don't think that has happened in many other scientific domains.

Dayan: You raise a very interesting example there with the advantage, inevitably, of looking over a long period. One looks backwards, and the point was made before about the EU's environmental programme starting in the early 1970s. At least from what I know, but I may be wrong, the United Nations' interest or activities in these areas, the International Agency Research on Cancer (IARC), the various UN-related bodies concerned with pesticides, like JMPR (Joint Meeting on Pesticide Residues of FAO and WHO), FAO (Food and Agriculture Organization), International Programme on Chemical Safety (IPCS), they all started I think in the 1960s, but their concentration at that time was exclusively, so far as I am aware, on human health. I am not sure how the environment, though very important, got into the scientific and political consciousness around those times.

Dr Peter Hunter: Could I just make one point about how the environment was regarded? There was a very substantial area of the world where the environment was regarded as a deadly, deadly enemy. In West Africa, for instance, there was a saying, 'Beware, beware the Bight of Benin/where few come out but many go in'.[44] This is a completely different and psychological and emotional view.

Berry: Can we go back to your point about methodology? Professor Dayan, you were asking about whether our capacity to do something serious in science depended on the methodology, which is a very important fundamental point. There is an interesting link here, I think, in looking at how opinion is formed. Celeste Condit in a very good review last year [2001] in *Nature Reviews in*

---

[43] The first important international conference on the assessment of the role of carbon dioxide and other greenhouse gases in climatic variations and associated impacts was held in Villach, Austria, in 1977. For details on climate change see www.wmo.ch/web/catalogue/New%20HTML/frame/engfil/wcn/wcn16.pdf (site accessed 11 February 2004). See also Last (1993).

[44] The Bight of Benin, a strip of land lying between the Volta and Lagos rivers in western Benin, acquired a reputation for dangerously high levels of malaria among European slave traders in the eighteenth century.

Genetics[45] analysed the way in which the public is influenced. The question of defining what constitutes 'the public' is quite a difficult one, and trying to obtain public opinion on xenotransplantation, for example, depends whether you are on the waiting list for a kidney or not. You are not going to get consensus views, but Condit has looked at how often opinions, frequently on the basis of indifferent science, make their way into legislation in the USA.

Her conclusion is that 'what gets said is what matters' and that much more influence is attributable to chat show hosts than to science (she produces a very good series of references to justify that assertion). This troubles me because, like you, I am concerned that our methodologies aren't good enough to measure what we sometimes draw conclusions about, and I deplore entirely the use of the precautionary principle, though it's much lauded in this field. The precautionary principle was the reason that I spent a great many years doing a lot of autopsies each year on sudden infant death syndrome [SIDS], because everybody knew it was sensible to sleep children on their front, because you nursed unconscious and immobile patients on their front.[46] In fact it killed them, and the change has been startling. In the last five years the SIDS rate has dropped from 1600 a year to lower than 400, of which about a quarter, unhappily, are known to be the result of criminal intervention.[47]

So there you have a precautionary principle, which seemed very rational but didn't have any science, but was enormously damaging. I share your reservations about some of the methodologies that we are using. I think that where we have got better at appreciating environmental risk it is because the methodology has improved, because we have a better idea of what are the indicator species, an ability that was almost entirely lacking 30 years ago. That's a very important consideration of how things have changed, or will change for the better scientifically. I think we make a better assessment of environmental impacts than we used to do.

---

[45] Condit (2001).

[46] Professor Sir Colin Berry wrote: 'As Chairman of the MRC Systems Board [Member 1988–90, Chairman 1990–92], I know the Council was under pressure to "do something" about SIDS. The problem is that there was nothing to do – there was no hypothesis to test. The first data on the position for sleeping came from Australia. See Beal and Blundell (1978); Fleming *et al.* (1990).' Letter to Dr Daphne Christie, 5 December 2003.

[47] Statistics for 2002 showed that sudden unexplained infant death in the UK decreased from 415 in 2001 to 342 in 2002, a drop of 17 per cent. Further statistics are given in *FSID News*, Magazine of the Foundation for the Study of Infant Deaths, Spring 2004, page 6. See also www.sids.org.uk/fsid/index.shtml (site accessed 9 December 2003).

Unfortunately I think public opinion often runs ahead of the science, as it has with sudden infant death. I believe it did after Hatfield too.[48] The ban on high-speed rail travel drove many more people back to the roads, and I am sure when the figures end up being analysed, we will see more people died as a consequence of that change. So leaping before you know is a dangerous thing to do, yet as a politician you have to leap! Yes, I think the point about the importance of the politics is absolutely central.

Woods: I think we have to be careful in relation to methodology. We have excellent chemical methodology and again speakers have alluded to the fact that we can both identify chemicals and detect very, very small amounts of them in various parts of the environment, including the human body. One of our great problems is that there has been no parallel between the development of chemical technology and analytical technology and the development of what are now called biomarkers of damage. Those two have not developed hand in hand. Therefore we are at the moment somewhat handicapped in linking up the presence of chemicals, the mechanism through which those chemicals may cause damage, and evidence that damage has occurred in whatever population, be it plant, animal or human.

Dayan: Could we just go a little bit further on that point? You can talk of analysis in terms of the ability to detect specific chemicals, which clearly has been absolutely vital, but it's only one very small factor in a picture. If you take a more analytical biological or ecological view you are likely to be more interested in populations, numbers, general health, reproductive health, turnover and so on. I am not an ecologist, and I wonder how well developed historically, for example, were ecological surveillance methods that could have been applied rationally way back in the 1960s or 1970s had the need for them been realized.

Lovelock: I think we suffered an unfortunate accident during the course of the twentieth century, and that was when ecology became dominated by a passionate

---

[48] On 17 October 2000 four people were killed and about 70 were injured when a GNER (Greater North Eastern Railway) train from King's Cross was derailed at Hatfield, about 16 miles north of London [Marston *et al.* (2000)]. A cracked and poorly maintained rail was subsequently discovered to be the cause, and many rail services were suspended or reduced for several months while the rail network was tested. No public enquiry was held into the crash, but 12 former employees of Network Rail and Railtrack, the companies responsible for track maintenance, were charged with manslaughter and offences under the Health and Safety legislation in July 2003. The companies themselves were also charged with corporate manslaughter.

interest in neo-Darwinism.[49] Although a most useful and valuable development of science, this caused biologists almost wholly to ignore the environment. It was a very theoretical topic, and all models made of populations of organisms were not transferable to the real world, and the tendency inclined to make the real world less interesting than models. This persisted right the way up to the 1990s and consequently we may have suffered a grievous loss of interest by competent biologists in the very questions that you have just raised.

Dayan: That would distract us into another theme of quantification and biology, but perhaps we had better not follow that black hole at the moment.

Professor Peter Farmer: I certainly agree with the comments of Professor Woods earlier, that the analytical technology has advanced far faster than our ability to detect biological effects resulting from the exposure, and I do agree that we have to understand the mechanisms and the scientific methods much better to be able to assess risks in these exposures, but I think there's a slight danger here that in a way the industrial analytical companies are pushing us forward faster than we are ready to go. Detection of a low amount of material does not necessarily mean that there's a risk associated with it, and I am afraid the public opinion is that if you can find it, there must be something nasty going on. So I do think we have to watch how we approach this problem, in getting down to measuring below femtograms, attograms, zeptograms of material,[50] less than one molecule per hundred cells of some toxic chemicals. We really have to think, 'What does it mean? Just because we can measure it, is it biologically significant or not?'

Dayan: In a sense that introduces an entirely new dimension into the broadest aspect of the development of chemicals in industrial use, let alone their release from natural sources. If you try to think back into the 1960s or the 1970s and

---

[49] Neo-Darwinism represents a synthesis of Charles Darwin's theory of evolution by natural selection and Gregor Mendel's genetic theory of inheritance [see Huxley (1942)]. It postulates that natural selection acts on the heritable genetic variations within individuals in populations, and the mutations provide the main source of these genetic variations [see Dawkins (1986); Dennett (1995)]. Because the genetic mutations seem to be rare, neo-Darwinism contends that evolution will be a slow, gradual process, and this has led to conflict with the 'punctuated equilibrium' model of evolution proposed in 1972 by Niles Eldridge and Stephen Jay Gould [Eldridge and Gould (1972)] which argues that evolutionary change happens quickly and in short bursts.

[50] A femtogram is 10^{-15} g, attogram 10^{-18} g, and zeptogram 10^{-21} g. See also note 14.

concepts like the dose–response curve[51] based on effects in human beings, or in other animals, we knew a certain amount, we knew ways of studying it of greater or lesser utility, but we had a concept, we had a philosophy, of how to investigate such matters. Until books like Rachel Carson's, until examples of problems occurring in the areas that could be very directly related to environmental contamination, until we had those examples, it's my impression that we didn't realize that there could even be problems on the scale that we are talking about. Now, was it only because the chemist could find organochloride residues all over the place, or were there other changes in the bases of the sciences that led us to realize what was going on? The fact was that we needed to study things more widely.

Professor Robert Smith: This is an opportunity to wander down memory lane. My memories of this go back to 1959–60, when my mentor at the time [Professor Richard Williams] had just published what became a classic text in toxicology called *Detoxication Mechanisms.*[52] This actually received very poor reviews at the time, and there was one particular review, published in the *Lancet*,[53] which said, 'Why would anyone have an interest in the fate of benzene?' That showed you the type of attitude, I think, that existed at the time, and I clearly remember someone in the office came to my desk and placed a copy of Rachel Carson's book upon my desk, and said, 'Bob, you should read this, this is important, because people will now be interested in the fate of chemicals in the environment,' which I think was quite a prescient thing to have said at the time of the attitudes towards toxicology. Clearly that was a very embryonic sign at the time.

But I do want to pick on one point, which was very nicely encapsulated by one of the earlier speakers, when he talked about numbers giving a spurious significance. I think that clearly Rachel Carson's book has had a tremendous effect, a positive effect in general, but it has had a down side, particularly when

---

[51] Dose–response curves are generated experimentally by exposing animals or tissue samples to varying concentrations of a substance and measuring its effect, or by examining effects in humans. This information can then be used to assess the pharmacological or toxicological impact of the substance. Some workers have claimed that such curves can be extrapolated to very low doses, implying that even at microlevels a toxicant retains its environmental effect. Others argue that each substance possesses a dose threshold (below which it is completely inactive) and therefore may be present in the environment at low levels without any adverse effect. See Moriarty (1988).

[52] Williams (1959).

[53] The review of the publication in the *Lancet* (1960) **i**: 684, gives no reference to benzene. Dr Christie has been unable to find this quote and Professor Robert Smith has not responded to a request for details.

her implications have been associated with our ability to measure and detect chemicals, and I think we still suffer the consequences of that now, 40 years later. It led to concepts such as vanishing zero and zero tolerance,[54] and I couldn't agree with you more about the damaging prospects of the precautionary principle we are having to live with now.

We still have to live with this problem of being able to detect these chemicals at minute levels but not place them into any sort of adequate risk–benefit analysis. My one hope about this is that this is now being counter-balanced by what I would call the 'biological toxicology' that has emerged in recent years, such as the BSE controversy and *Escherichia coli*.[55] I think these toxic effects attributable to infections are now putting toxicology – I emphasize chemical toxicology – into a proper perspective. But my main concern now is the way in which zero tolerance and the precautionary principle really has emerged in this whole debate, and I think it has been very damaging for the entire question of chemical technology.

Johnson: Following on from that last point and again an anecdotal perspective: I can very much remember in 1974–75 negotiating through the European Commission and then through the Council, the first EU directives on water quality.[56] I think it makes the point that these were very mechanistical-type directives, they had 60 or 70 parameters and with lots of numbers in them. Of course, the politicians were extremely thrilled to be able to agree to numbers, because when it came to the Council it looked hard, it looked forceful, and they were able to say, 'We have got a clear numerical EU standard'. But if I go back to the Working Groups, on which, of course, governments were represented and usually chaired at Commission level (although at Council it was a Council representative), it was a much more haphazard exercise altogether. Just picking up, for example, the value of nitrates in water: you know we went round the table and various people said it should be 100 ppm [parts per million], 1000 ppm, and finally the difference was split.[57]

---

[54] Dr Robert Flanagan wrote: 'The concept is that "if it can be measured it must be harmful".' E-mail to Dr Daphne Christie, 29 March 2004. See Carson (1962): 165–7.

[55] See www.fsis.usda.gov/OPHS/ecolrisk/prelim.htm (site accessed 12 March 2004).

[56] For water policy in the European Union see, for example, www.europa.eu.int/comm/environment/water/ (site accessed 11 December 2003).

[57] Mr Stanley Johnson wrote: 'Council Directive of 16 June 1975, "Quality requirements for surface water intended for the abstraction of drinking water", specified a recommended value of 25 mg/l and an imperative value of 50 mg/l for the presence of nitrates in water.' Note on draft transcript, 12 December 2003.

This may seem all very funny and of course in those days why did you have a value of the nitrate at all in water? It was to make the point that has already been made, a purely health-related value. The idea was that you avoided the blue-baby syndrome[58] and so on and so forth, but we paid the price, I think, later on. If you have been picking up the papers in the last few days and if you looked at the letters in *The Times* or the *Telegraph* this morning,[59] you will see that farmers all over England are now protesting at the enormous expense that is going to be imposed on the farming industry in its efforts to come to terms with the revised nitrate rules. I think the issue that we have to ask ourselves is how many of these standards were adopted because the numbers were there, because the measurements were there, and were justified in health or ecological terms? It's rather frightening to me now when you see the billions, literally billions of pounds [sterling] that were involved in implementing the nitrates directive, money that could possibly have been spent somewhere else. It's slightly worrying to me that we went down that route too quickly and perhaps too light-heartedly.

While I have the floor I wanted to pick up a point that Professor Lovelock made. How have we moved on from seeing the definition of standards purely in health terms, to seeing them also in a wider environmental context? He did mention the chlorofluorocarbon (CFC) and ozone issue, and I think it is a brilliant issue to bring to the floor at this point, because of course once you started defining standards on ozone and on CFC releases, it was not only because of the impact on health, it was for much wider concerns altogether. If we are talking environmental toxicology in the largest sense, the overwhelming argument in front of the world is what are the values for the presence of greenhouse gases in the atmosphere that we are going to be ready to tolerate? Is it twice the pre-industrial level; is it three times the pre-industrial level? Those of course are not going to be health-related arguments; they are going to be arguments in the widest ecological context.

---

[58] Nitrates oxidize haemoglobin to methaemoglobin which cannot bind with oxygen, so the overall oxygen-carrying capacity of the blood is reduced. Infants are more susceptible than adults. Blue-baby syndrome is the name given to nitrate poisoning in neonates. The disease can be caused by intake of water and vegetables high in nitrate, or exposure to chemicals containing nitrate. Groundwater gets contaminated by leaching of nitrate generated from fertilizer used on agricultural land, and waste dumps in rural and urban areas. Further details are provided in a note from Mr Stanley Johnson to Dr Daphne Christie, 12 December 2003.

[59] 12 March 2002. The EU directive restricted the amount of manure farmers were allowed to spread within nitrate-vulnerable zones. At least 10 000 farmers were forced to transport millions of tonnes of manure across many miles. See Uhlig (2002).

Lovelock: One reminiscence that has bothered me all through my life's work in environmental chemistry is the passionate interest of the public in anything that might be a carcinogen. The media know full well that if you want to tell a good environmental story, bring out its carcinogenic significance. I think concern over stratospheric ozone depletion began when it was realized that malignant melanoma might be connected with it.[60] So I ask, is the public's fear and perception of cancer doing us all a great deal of harm? And shouldn't more be said to take people's minds away from that kind of feared end-stage, instead of making it appear to be of major public importance?

Berry: I think this is really a very important point. The public perception depends entirely on where the public is led, and I think it is often misled. The example I think you know I always take is soya protein, which is always said to be terribly good for you, and to stop you getting menopausal symptoms. This has led to people feeding male infants soya formulae, rather than cow's milk-based formulae, giving them levels of plasma oestriol that are 13–20 000-times the normal values.[61] There's a very good study from Jean Golding in Bristol[62] that has shown that vegetarian mothers produce male infants with a very high incidence of hypospadias. This is an entirely predictable scientific effect, yet still soya proteins always get a good press, though genistein,[63] one of the principal phyto-oestrogens in them, is carcinogenic in Professor Lovelock's definition – that is, DNA-altering in appropriate circumstances.[64]

That's the sort of thing that the press usually calls a carcinogen, though that's a naive approach to the subject, but nevertheless that's what happens. So here you have a human teratogen and almost certainly a human carcinogen in some views. I don't believe that at all, but you know it could be presented in that way. Yet it is something that every 'foodie' presents in their newspaper pages as being terribly good for you. So I think a lot of public opinion is led by a non-science-based process, and I do think that that can be damaging. Look at the sperm count nonsense and the changes that were attributed to all sorts of things. Enormous

---

[60] For a review see Amron and Moy (1991). See also Advisory Group on the Medical Aspects of Air Pollution Episodes (1991).

[61] Setchell *et al.* (1997).

[62] North and Golding (2000).

[63] See Kulling *et al.* (1999); De Lemos (2001).

[64] Professor Anthony Dayan wrote: 'Genistein is not regarded as genotoxic by many.' Note on draft transcript, 28 November 2003.

efforts were made in the scientific community to devise new animal tests that might or might not have a predictive value. I think it was about as much a non-event as nitrate was in drinking water, and again costing huge sums of money.

Dayan: Professor Carter, you have been at the hinge of carcinogenicity debates for many years, subjected to pressures on all sides.

Carter: I have two general comments to make at this stage. As people have said already, public perceptions of problems such as carcinogenicity are often manipulated in directions that are anything but soundly based science. Secondly, scientific results are often indifferently presented to the general public. Furthermore, there is understandable confusion when the public hears apparently familiar words, such as 'hazard' and 'risk', being used in specialized ways. Distinctions between 'hazard' and 'risk' are not widely appreciated by the general public, and similar difficulties arise with other words and concepts that scientists and regulators may use.

Professor Robert Maynard: Chairman, I think it's important that scientists shouldn't transfer blame directly to the public for getting things wrong. Scientists are largely to blame for the scares that spread among the public. We are all aware of publications before the data are solid, publications that have been made to try to produce the next grant application. Sir Colin Berry drew attention to this recently in a publication,[65] and these are what the media pick up. We should know by now, and God knows we have had enough evidence of it, that the media exists to find things to entertain and amuse and worry the public. Scientists exist to obtain grants to continue their curious activities. Those two groups will feed off each other, and so much of the blame, I think, for scares about carcinogenicity problems does lie with part of the scientific community, not only with the media or the public.

Dayan: May we follow that a bit further, because I think it raises some really quite fascinating general issues? A lot of the carcinogenicity debate was set off and driven by an American Congressman, Thomas Delaney. The famous Delaney Clause in 1958,[66] embodied the notion that anything that was shown to be carcinogenic, by

[65] Berry (2002).

[66] Professor Anthony Dayan wrote: 'In 1958 Thomas Delaney proposed and the US Congress accepted an amendment to the US Food, Drug and Cosmetic Bill, which passed into US law in 1958. It broadly stated that any chemical found to be carcinogenic in laboratory animals or humans should not be added to the US food supply.' Note on draft transcript, 28 November 2003. See also page 25 and Tansey and Reynolds (1997).

any sort of experiment, should not be permitted in anything that the US public would be exposed to in foods and other materials in common use. An enormous amount of money was then devoted to investigating the causes and treatment of cancer. This was not so long before Nixon's war against cancer,[67] which was all going to be won before he finished his second term in office, wasn't it?

There was a huge pressure against cancer at that time, partly perhaps reflecting the ability of the medical profession to diagnose it more effectively, and the beginnings of rational and moderately effective cancer treatments. Maybe it's understandable why, but can we try to place ourselves in a different position? If one were starting out now with the sort of problems that we have been touching on, but without today's knowledge, are there lessons that we can draw that would show us how to learn, how to appreciate? It's really about appreciating the unknown, allowing for the unknown in future, but without, as you very rightly said, being scared. The precautionary principle is a marvellous excuse for doing absolutely nothing.

Woods: There is one thing, Mr Chairman, which perhaps we could do if we were to start again. I am using that very dangerous diagnostic instrument, the retrospectroscope, which is only used at maximum magnification, and huge illumination. This question concerns decisions made by those who advise legislators, made not in secret but certainly in closed sessions. If I had my time again, I would like to see much more openness. Some, but not all of the problems that we are seeing now about the interpretation of science and the way in which science is purveyed to the public in relation to their own interests and in their own environment and lives (I think there are others – this has been written on quite extensively) derive from the fact that some of the discussions were held behind closed doors. I have been very impressed recently in various ways in the Committee on Toxicity that I have been chairing until very recently, about open discussion of these matters. I suspect that if there had been more open discussion about some of the matters that affect the environment then some of the concerns and worries, certainly in the public perception, would not be there.

Maynard: The point about openness, Mr Chairman, is a very good one and Professor Woods is right to raise it. Open discussion is a laudable aim, but the way in which government is conducted is limited by staff resources and the amount of money that the public is prepared to have the government spend on

---

[67] Professor Anthony Dayan added: 'In 1971 President Richard Nixon initiated a "War on Cancer" and greatly increased funding for research and treatment.' Note on draft transcript, 28 November 2003.

its behalf. It's difficult to reach sensible decisions at the best of times when the data are limited, the interpretation is a bit varied, and the number of experts that you can call upon for an independent opinion is small. To try to reach a sensible decision, and to sustain that decision in front of hostile criticism – and some of it was deliberately hostile – would simply make the decision-making process more difficult. Now I have taken an extreme view there, as people will recognize, but it is designed to prompt discussion.

Carter: Just to pick up one point, Chairman, about chronology. *Silent Spring* was published in 1962. The Delaney amendment, I think, was promulgated in 1958.[68] Work on genotoxic and nongenotoxic mechanisms in carcinogenesis began in the late 1960s and developed rapidly thereafter.[69] I think these dates help to place Rachel Carson's book in a historical and also a scientific context.

Dayan: Perhaps partly because the concept of carcinogenesis, the mechanisms and the ability to test for the potential of carcinogenicity of something in certain ways, these came together in a practicable way at about that sort of time and it became feasible.[70] For reproductive toxicity, on the other hand, there were either some relatively very simple things like teratogenicity testing – forgive me, Professor Berry, but it is relatively simple – whereas the complexities of the full reproductive process and the influences on it were (and still are) really much less well understood. Certainly in terms of devising regimes for studying the propensity of compounds to have relevant effects, that would be and is, I think, far more difficult.

Carter: As far as carcinogenic mechanisms are concerned, genotoxic effects can now be predicted and demonstrated with a reasonable degree of accuracy.[71] But there is an uncomfortable disparity here with our poor understanding of many nongenotoxic processes. The latter are likely to predominate when it comes to thinking of carcinogenic contributions from the environment for human populations.

---

[68] See note 66.

[69] Professor Richard Carter wrote: 'See, for example, *Monographs on the Evaluation of Carcinogenic Risks to Humans*, an ongoing series published by the International Agency for Research in Cancer (IARC), 1972–, Lyon, vols 1–80. The results of short-term mutagenicity tests were routinely included in these monographs after 1974.' Note on draft transcript, 1 December 2003.

[70] Professor Anthony Dayan wrote: 'A great advance was the formal acceptance of genetic toxicity testing in the early 1980s as a valid indicator of the carcinogenic risk of chemicals.' Note on draft transcript, 28 November 2003. See Ashby *et al.* (1988).

[71] McGregor *et al.* (1999).

Smith: I think we should complete the sequence of events, which began with Rachel Carson's book and then the Delaney amendment, and then came the NTP [National Toxicology Program] for the evaluation of chemical carcinogenicity,[72] which has done far more harm than good in my opinion. This is really a role, not of science, but of biopolitics, where the mission is to discover carcinogens through a very extreme process of testing. There is a mission to uncover carcinogens, because it relates to the future of the funding process, and many are left years later trying to deal with the consequences of looking at the results of these test programmes, where chemicals are being tested under very unreal conditions, which have little or no relationship to the actual conditions of use.

Berry: We might go back to the point made earlier about animal use. I think these programmes have materially affected people's attitudes to the use of animals in research, because many of them are quite clearly nonsensical studies, as you have said, 'That's a misuse of animals'. A lot of ecological studies require the use of animals in a very obvious way, because you are looking at the whole biological system. I think carcinogenicity studies, perhaps in the doses that have been used particularly in the NTP, are the least informative, in terms of science, and the most damaging, in terms of the misuse of animals.[73] I don't believe we are going to be able to devise systems that won't depend on animals in some part, and I do believe we have to be much more cautious about how they are used. I agree that the NTP was a very bad example of use of animals.

Dayan: In terms of predicting genotoxic potential in the field of carcinogenesis, we rightly associate the name of Professor Bruce Ames with a suite of very good test methods for certain purposes.[74] Professor Ames has probably spent as much time and certainly as much personal effort as anyone on discussing the problems of naturally occurring carcinogens, but we never ever talk about it, we never hear

---

[72] The National Toxicology Program (NTP) was established in 1978 by the US Department of Health and Human Services (DHHS) to coordinate toxicological testing programmes within the Department, to strengthen the science base in toxicology; to develop and validate improved testing methods; and to provide information about potentially toxic chemicals to health regulatory and research agencies, the scientific and medical communities, and the public. Its headquarters are at the National Institutes of Health's National Institute of Environmental Health Sciences (NIEHS) located in Research Triangle Park, North Carolina.

[73] See, for example, Sharpe (1988): 104–5.

[74] Professor Anthony Dayan added: 'Professor Ames developed simple and reliable methods for detecting many types of genotoxic activity of chemicals in the bacterium *Salmonella typhimurium*.' Note on draft transcript, 28 November 2003. See Ames *et al.* (1973); Ashby *et al.* (1988).

about them. Why not? Are we not as worried by selenium as we are by sulphur something-or-the-other from the chemical world? We have a very warped outlook. Still, we don't want to go too far down that road.

May I raise another issue? Many of us have had contact with industry in one-way or the other. In the area that we are discussing, one could look at industry in two different ways: one is to say that industry will do whatever it has to do in order to get its products used, and where appropriate, registered, so it will follow requirements rather than setting them. I think that's rather a disparaging view of the better scientific companies, and in many instances they have led the research that has shown the way certainly to the delineation of genuine hazards and of the means to predict them. In this context of environmental toxicology where has industry been, what have they been doing? Have they simply followed?

Lovelock: You anticipated me on this one. I had the good fortune in, I think it was 1963, to be taken on as an adviser to Lord Rothschild when he was science coordinator for Shell.[75] In addition, this was just after Rachel Carson's book had appeared. He was furious with her for what he thought was overstating the case, but it was significant that Shell chemists were among the very first to start measuring pesticides in all sorts of things, even before Rachel Carson's book appeared. I think it was not long afterwards that industry responded by taking dieldrin and aldrin out of production before they were actually banned.[76] I think industry often gets a very bad name – it just happens to suit the way the politics or the media or whatever, I don't know who's to blame, but it always happens that way. The same happened with the CFC affair.[77] The response of industry

---

[75] Professor James Lovelock wrote: 'Lord Rothschild called me to his office in the Shell Centre, London, in July 1963. He said that he had just heard that I had given up paid employment and intended to practise science independently. He then offered me a retainer of £1500 a year to think in my spare time about the science problems confronting Shell. I accepted his offer with gratitude, for it enabled me to break all my ties and start doing science from my home laboratory.' Letter to Dr Daphne Christie, 9 December 2003.

[76] From the 1950s until 1970, aldrin and dieldrin were widely used as pesticides to protect crops like corn and cotton. The EPA banned all their uses in 1974, except for the control of termites and, in 1987, they were banned completely. See also note 13.

[77] Professor James Lovelock wrote: 'It was discovered in 1973 by Sherwood Rowlands and Mario Molina that the stratospheric ozone layer was in danger of depletion from the presence of chlorine-containing organic compounds such as the CFCs and industrial solvents such as methyl chloroform. Soon afterwards political activists used this information as a weapon to attack the chemical industry and long before the true extent of the danger was scientifically established newspaper headlines carried statements such as, "Spray cans will destroy all life on Earth". These wild exaggerations were almost never properly challenged by scientists or by industry representatives.' Letter to Dr Daphne Christie, 9 December 2003.

there I think was magnificent. They accepted that there was a danger and set about preparing alternatives that would not be so risky. I don't think that the Montreal protocol[78] would ever have been agreed had not industry been so supportive, but they are always portrayed as the bad men, the wicked ones.

Hunter: Can I please just add a comment in there? The aerosol manufacturers in this country couldn't believe it, they thought all their birthdays had come at once when they had to substitute butane for CFCs, something that they never thought they were allowed to put in a domestic product, and their bank balances were assured for the next 20 years.[78a]

Johnson: Just on the CFC point. I don't think one should overestimate the altruism of industry. I do remember there was a very, very active industrial lobby in the mid-1970s, against the findings that seemed to be coming out of the USA on the CFC issue. The USA regulated their use of CFCs long before the EU did,[79] and certainly companies like ICI were very reluctant to move down that route. I would say that it was probably only when, I think it was in 1983, Joe Farman of the British Antarctic Survey [BAS] incontrovertibly spotted the ozone hole[80] and so on that UK industry, or European industry, really came into line wholeheartedly; that's my impression on the CFC issue.

---

[78] Professor James Lovelock wrote: 'In 1987 representatives from over 100 nations met in Montreal to sign a protocol banning the manufacture and emission of the chlorofluorocarbons (CFCs) so as to prevent the further erosion of the stratospheric ozone layer due to their presence in the atmosphere.' Letter to Dr Daphne Christie, 9 December 2003.

[78a] Dr Robert Flanagan wrote: 'Butane is purified liquefied petroleum gas consisting of propane, isobutane and butane. It is available cheaply in large quantity but is flammable hence prior to the requirement to find a cheap non-CFC aerosol propellant had not been considered safe for this application. There have been fires attributed to domestic use of butane-containing aerosols [see, for example, Marc *et al.* (2001)].' E-mail to Dr Daphne Christie, 29 March 2004.

[79] Toxic Substances Control Act, 1976.

[80] Mr Stanley Johnson wrote: 'Having gained his degree from the University of Cambridge, Joseph Farman was appointed as a scientific officer to the Falkland Islands Dependencies Survey – the forerunner of the British Antarctic Survey (BAS). After two winters he returned to the UK and became Head of the Geophysics Section of BAS and a senior research fellow with the University of Edinburgh, to which the Section was affiliated. Moving back to Cambridge in 1976 to the newly built BAS headquarters, Joseph Farman held a variety of job titles from Head of the Stratosphere Section to Head of Chemistry, Radiation and Dynamics. It was he who provided the critical link between ozone and chlorofluorocarbons (CFCs) in the now famous *Nature* paper of 1985 [Farman *et al.* (1985)].' Note on draft transcript, 12 December 2003.

Corcoran: In addition to legislation on pesticides there is also extensive legislation on new and existing industrial chemicals brought on to the European market.[81] Extensive testing is required both for mammalian toxicology and for ecotoxicology, but one must always remember the economic dimension. It costs money to do tests and to assess them and you have to make a balance between the likely benefit of the product, the likely risks, and the costs of the whole assessment process both to industry and government. In 1999 the UK government published a strategy statement on chemicals, which proposed a duty of care for the chemical industry.[82] This could be summed up as saying that manufacturers shouldn't simply wait until a test is demanded by regulators, but when they produce a product they should take responsibility for thinking of what its effects may be both to human health and the environment. They should carry out the necessary testing and make their own judgement about how the product should be marketed, or if it should be marketed at all.

But we have been talking largely about Western industry. Remember what happened with the organochlorine pesticides. Some were banned in developed countries many years ago,[83] but DDT and other organophosphate pesticides continued to be manufactured in large quantities in the developing world (in India and China, for example) because the process is well understood, the materials are quite cheap and easy to manufacture, are usually off-patent, and, being persistent also makes them very effective in some ways. Persistence in a chemical does have its downside in terms of environmental risks, but it can also make it more effective. For these reasons, DDT and other persistent chemicals continue to be manufactured in the developing world.

Dayan: Peter, you have brought out a point indirectly: you referred to the European Commission system for notification of chemicals and the need to follow particular regimes of study, of protocols for mammalian testing, environmental testing, and the physical hazards as well. What led to the selection of the particular types of experimentation if you know it? Not so much the

---

[81] Dr Peter Corcoran wrote: 'The relevant EU legislation is Directive 67/548/EEC (sometimes known as the sixth amendment) for new chemicals, and Regulation 793/93 for existing chemicals.' Letter to Dr Daphne Christie, 24 November 2003. See www.europe.osha.eu.int/legislation/directives/ (site accessed 2 December 2003).

[82] Department of the Environment, Transport and Regions (1999).

[83] See, for example, note 76.

detail, but the purposes for which those experiments were done? Who decided? Was it the scientists, the politicians, and was industry involved?

Corcoran: The test protocols and testing packages were decided by committees of scientists from government, the public sector, industry and from academia.

Johnson: As far as the toxicological tests were concerned, I would say that we did rely to a very large extent on the work that came out of the OECD [Organization for Economic Cooperation and Development] and this was taken over into the EU as the basis, for example, of the 1967 sixth amendment[84] which dealt with the question of new chemicals coming on to the market. Here the issue of course was to try to agree a system also with the USA because the USA had their ToSCA[85] regulation, which was somewhat different in concept to the system the EU was putting into place. One of the intriguing things now, of course, and I think this seminar is very timely, is that the EU has taken upon itself to reassess the toxicity, including environmental toxicity, of thousands and thousands of existing chemicals, chemicals that are already on the market, which have not so far been evaluated.[86] Of course the danger from this exercise is almost incalculable if it is driven by the zero-tolerance philosophy.

Berry: I was just going to say in response to Peter Corcoran's point that I think that many of the tests were done because they could be done. There was a desire to measure something about the environment and here was, say, something you could do with fish, or something you could do with mites, and because it could be done, it was chosen to be the test that you did, much as mutagenicity in the Ames test was chosen at that time because it was suddenly a methodology that was available.[87] It goes back to your point, that the methodology often drives these testing programmes, simply because if there's no way of studying it you can't do anything.

---

[84] See note 81. Mr Stanley Johnson wrote: 'In 1979, the sixth amending directive to the Council directive of 1967 on the classification, packaging and labelling of dangerous substances introduced compulsory prior notification of any new chemicals placed on the market.' Note on draft transcript, 12 December 2003.

[85] The Toxic Substances Control Act (ToSCA) of 1976 authorized the Environmental Protection Agency (EPA) to obtain data from industry on health and environmental effects of chemical substances and mixtures. See note 79.

[86] Draft legislation to implement the Registration, Evaluation and Authorization of Chemicals (REACH) Policy, of the European Commission Environmental Directive. Further details can be found at www.chemicalspolicy.org/docu.euni.shtml (site accessed 3 March 2004).

[87] Ames *et al.* (1979).

Dayan: I wonder historically how this arose, the trialkyltins, such as tributyltin [TBT], are very powerful compounds for certain purposes. They were widely used at one time, weren't they, for painting the bottoms of ships, as antifouling agents?[88] Ultimately the realization came that these agents were leaching into the seawater, and having unexpected and quite disastrous effects on various forms of marine life. How did that chain of evidence accrue, how did it start?

Corcoran: I think I know the answer to that one. It's because of the French concern about oysters. The French take their oysters very seriously, so when oysters started to get misshapen, the shells started to thicken and they became less palatable, the French started to look for reasons and they quickly lighted on TBT as the cause. They then applied pressure on other EU member states, who perhaps didn't take their oysters quite so seriously, to do something about it. So I think it was direct observation, backed up by laboratory experiments.

Dayan: A nice example, in the negative sense, of the problems of releasing a chemical where it can enter the environment with virtually no knowledge of its possible environmental consequences.

Dr Dennis Simms: Could I add to what Peter Corcoran has just said? It produced the largest correspondence that we in our division [Toxic Substances Division in the Department of the Environment] ever had. The boating industry took a very dim view of any attempt to deal with TBT and it took far longer than it should have done to be banned, simply because of the weight of the correspondence we received. It scared everybody in the department.

Dr Robert Flanagan: It is interesting in view of previous discussions about some perceived problems being method led, because the unravelling of the TBT story was entirely observational. We could not measure TBT itself at the concentrations attained in biological systems until relatively recently, and perhaps one reason it took so long to piece the story together was because there wasn't the analytical methodology there to help provide the objective evidence as to what was happening.

Smith: This is a slight change of direction, Chairman, and it's rather a mundane point as well, but we are talking about the legacies of Rachel Carson. I think we

---

[88] Professor Anthony Dayan wrote: 'To prevent the growth of algae and small crustacea that adhered to the hulls of ships, resulting in increased resistance to movement and great fuel consumption [see Barnes and Stoner (1959)].' Note on draft transcript, 28 November 2003. TBT stops the growth and lowers the fuel consumption.

shouldn't forget the enormous impact her book and its consequences had on the educational establishments, because numerous degrees and MSc programmes came into play. In its heyday, environmental science, in particular toxicology, had the equivalent of the impact on business of IT at the present time. The other thing we should mention is that in many ways it was the salvation of chemistry in UK universities. Chemistry departments were in severe decline through lack of students, and many chemistry departments got into bed with environmental sciences, and this, in fact, has been the salvation of chemistry. I think we shouldn't lose sight of this point, Mr Chairman, the important impact upon academia and its effect upon the continuity of chemistry.

Dayan: An interesting aspect, yes. We are going to cite another incident in the history of the environment and toxicology, which in some textbooks of toxicology and environmental law is given as much prominence as TBT and oysters. This was Seveso,[89] with the release of dioxins over a large area and its dramatic consequences.[90] Now there had been dioxins released before with effects, and subsequently, though perhaps none of them on quite that scale.[91] But disregarding for the moment the EEC Seveso directive,[92] because that came much later, for all sorts of reasons and not all of them creditable either, I think. How important was Seveso really in setting off another aspect of understanding of environmental toxicology?

---

[89] The Seveso accident happened in 1976 at a chemical plant manufacturing pesticides and herbicides. A dense vapour cloud containing tetrachlorodibenzoparadioxin (TCDD, commonly known as dioxin) was released from a reactor, used for the production of trichlorophenol, Dioxin is a poisonous and carcinogenic by-product of an uncontrolled exothermic reaction. Although no immediate fatalities were reported, kilogram quantities of the substance lethal to humans even in microgram doses were widely dispersed, which resulted in an immediate contamination of some ten square miles of land and vegetation. More than 600 people had to be evacuated from their homes and as many as 2000 were treated for dioxin poisoning. Further details can be found at http://europa.eu.int/comm/environment/seveso/#2 (site accessed 23 July 2003). See also Fuller (1977).

[90] Professor Anthony Dayan wrote: 'There has since been continuing uncertainty about the possible effects of the exposure on the residents with claims of birth defects, mental retardation and many types of cancer in people, and some possible effects on grazing animals there.' Note on draft transcript, 28 November 2003.

[91] See, for example, International Agency for Research on Cancer (IARC) (1997). See also McGregor *et al.* (1998).

[92] Professor Anthony Dayan wrote: 'An EC Directive intended to control the safety of large chemical plants which might present a major threat to public safety if there were an accident; Council Directive 82/501/EC.' Note on draft transcript, 28 November 2003.

Berry: There wasn't much understanding, I wouldn't have thought. It set off an epidemiological study.[93] I was just thinking that it demonstrated another methodological point, the practical point that there was suddenly thought to be an increase in human malformations there, but there had been inadequate ascertainment before and the malformation rate hadn't changed. It's interesting how those myths live on. With the same sort of issue, with regard to 2,4,5-T [2, 4, 5-trichlorophenoxyacetic acid] in Vietnam, the anti-Vietnam war feeling in the USA spilled over into the Agent Orange issue.[94] I took part in the 2,4,5-T review that Robert Kilpatrick chaired,[95] and I always remember his saying that the only way you could die from the effects of 2,4,5-T was to fall into a barrel of it and drown.[95a] But that didn't affect the important fact that you knew that it wasn't the commercial-grade 2,4,5-T that was being used in Vietnam, it was a higher-level, dioxin-contaminated compound. You can't have that kind of discussion in public. I think that since dioxins have become a bad word and are going to stay with us forever in the public mind, I don't think there's a dioxin desensitization programme that's going to work.

Johnson: To answer your question, Chairman, about Seveso. My recollection was that the accident was sometime in the summer of 1976, and I remember having to go to Milan about three days after the accident.[96] I think at that stage I was responsible in the European Commission for that side of activities, and while we were there we tried to see what lessons could be learnt for EU environmental policy at that time. I think it moved the EU in two directions. In a most immediate sense it moved it in the direction of adopting the directive on major industrial accidents, accidents coming from major industrial plants, and led to an interest in industrial emissions and pollutants coming out of chimney stacks.

So that was one major thrust. Later on, of course, we can see various other directives that have attempted to regulate emissions from industry. But the other area, and this is what I think you meant when you referred to the Seveso directive, is that people

---

[93] See Fuller (1977).

[94] Gough (1986).

[95] Thomas M. (1997). See also www-green.cusu.cam.ac.uk/archive/a700y/pesticid.htm (site accessed 9 December 2003).

[95a] Dr Robert Flanagan wrote: 'Dr Kilpatrick was talking about topical exposure to the diluted formulation. The commercial concentrate and even the diluted formulation can kill if ingested.' E-mail to Dr Daphne Christie, 29 March 2004.

[96] See note 89.

now more or less refer to the Seveso directive as being the EU directive on the movement of toxic waste around the Community. This was spurred on by concerns about what to do with the, I think, 40 barrels of toxic waste, the legacy of the clean up at ICMESA [Industrie Chimiche Mendionali Società Azionaria].[97] I would say that you are right because this did shift the EU's environmental policy towards taking much more seriously (a) the whole question of toxic waste, and (b) the general question of the disposal of waste, and I think we are seeing this today with the 'fridge mountain' issue.[98] If you want to look at these milestones, I think you would be absolutely right to say that within the EU, Seveso was one such milestone.

There were a couple of others, by the way. There was a tanker spill off the coast of Brittany, the *Amoco Cadiz* incident.[99] This led to a new policy dimension, which was the extent you could try to deal with pollution resulting from oil spills at sea, which is another form of pollution, like contamination, which we haven't talked about yet today but is worth thinking about. The other major milestone, was Bhopal, which didn't occur within the EU but had a colossal impact on people's thinking. Here was a US company, not an EU company, Union Carbide, being implicated in an accident which led to the death of maybe 3–4000 people with a number of longer-term consequences.[100] Yes, I think you are absolutely right that these discrete events have had a terrific impact in making environmental policy. Whether it moves in the right direction is another matter.

Dayan: Before you leave that point – I am sorry, I don't want to pick on you but you have very special knowledge in that area – why is it that those events that you have mentioned have had such a dramatic impact, whereas the fact that the

[97] See eco-informa.ead.anl.gov/abstracts/110xF_Fortunati.pdf (site accessed 12 March 2004). Further details are provided in a note from Mr Stanley Johnson to Dr Daphne Christie, 12 December 2003.

[98] The UK disposed of unwanted fridges by sending them to giant metal crushers that released CFCs. Under new EU regulations, fridges have to be crushed in special closed units, which captured the CFCs in liquid form so that they could then be burned and destroyed. However, because the UK didn't have any of the new recycling plants in place, thousands of fridges piled up, hence the term 'fridge mountain'. Mr Stanley Johnson wrote: 'The problem arose in the UK with the entry into force of EU Council Regulation 2037/2000 regarding the removal of ozone depleting substances (ODS) prior to disposal.' Note on draft transcript, 12 December 2003.

[99] Mr Stanley Johnson wrote: 'The *Amoco Cadiz* ran aground off the coast of Brittany, France, on 16 March 1978, spilling 68.7 million gallons of oil. It is currently number 6 on the list of the largest oil spills of all time.' Note on draft transcript, 12 December 2003.

[100] On 3 December 1984 methyl isocyanate gas leaked from a Union Carbide India Limited (UCIL) pesticide plant in Bhopal, India, just after midnight. Further details can be found at www.bhopal.com/ (site accessed 23 July 2003). See Tansey (1993).

Po Valley in Italy has been heavily contaminated with pesticides for 15 years and nothing was done except to allow the Italians to announce on the international stage what they were going to do, but never actually got round to doing?[101] The EC was well aware of it, because it had been passing exemptions from its own regulations on a regular basis for decades.

Johnson: I am not quite sure I remember these exemptions for the Po Valley as such. It might be that we didn't know what was going on, which is perhaps another matter.

Dayan: There was serious abuse of atrazine, paraquat and other herbicides by Italian farmers. The drinking water obtained from the Po river water contained many such substances.

Johnson: It does raise another whole issue altogether, which is what you might call the implementation issue, and, no, we don't want to get into that now, but it's a jolly important issue. We can have any amount of legislation, but the next step is implementation.

Woods: There is one other aspect of Seveso, and that is that a prospective study of the population was set up which is still going on.[102] One of the problems that advisory committees face, as you may well know, Chairman, is that many of the data with which we are presented are not proper prospective studies, they are often retrospective, and they are often on very small populations, and very often rather badly done.

I wanted to pick up on a point made earlier about the presentation of results. I think it was Bob Maynard who asked what use is made of those results?[103] Not only are scientific results presented indifferently to the public at large, they are also presented without criticism of the quality of the science that lay behind the writing of the paper. We see this time and time again. Conclusions in the scientific literature that are used by various organizations – pressure groups, individuals – to press a particular point, when, if you properly analyse the nature of that evidence, the science behind it is of a very poor quality.

---

[101] Professor Anthony Dayan wrote: 'Very heavy use of pesticides for many years in the Po Valley resulted in extensive contamination of drinking and other water supplies there. In the 1980s the Italian government repeatedly obtained the agreement of the EC to supply water that contained pesticides at levels exceeding the limits in the Drinking Water Directive (1987).' Note on draft transcript, 28 November 2003.

[102] Pesatori *et al.* (2003).

[103] See page 23.

Dayan: Alar was a very good example of that.[104]

Maynard: Chairman, may I return to the point that Frank Woods has just drawn attention to again. That's the need for the very careful examination of the evidence and I am dubious that in areas that have attracted a high public profile, you can get that cold, careful examination of the evidence while you are under intense public pressure. There's no desire to conceal here, but it's the difficulty of conducting a discussion when a large part of the audience have already reached a conclusion.

Pat Lawther, who was invited but was unable to be here today, made this point some time ago when he was conducting the inquiry into the toxic effects of environmental lead on children.[105] He said that every morning as he walked through the two lines of protesters he had babies shaken in his face. He said that it was so difficult to face the possibility of reaching a decision that would obviously be unpalatable to the majority. The difficulty that all expert committees face is that sometimes you may have to sum up and conclude dead against what the public or at least the vociferous part of the public hope you will conclude. That's really difficult to do, and to protect advisers from abuse is terribly important, otherwise governments will not be able to attract advisers of sufficient quality. What we will attract are people of enormous courage, of course, but not necessarily enormous ability; the two don't always go together.

Dayan: That's why we are very thankful to have people of your stature that we can shelter behind.

Hunter: There's one other major environmental toxic accident that occurred when mercury got into seawater in Japan, causing Minamata disease.[106]

---

[104] Professor Anthony Dayan wrote: 'Alar is a hydrazine derivative used in the cultivation of apples. Media stories that it was an animal carcinogen under certain circumstances had grave effects for a time on the sale and consumption of apples in the early 1990s.' Note on draft transcript, 28 November 2003.

[105] Department of Health and Social Security, Working Party on Lead in the Environment (1980). See also Lansdown and Yule (1986).

[106] Minamata is a small factory town dominated by the Chisso Corporation, facing the Shiranui Sea. The Chisso Corporation started as a fertilizer and carbide company, later producing petrochemicals and plastics. From 1932 to 1968, it dumped an estimated 27 tonnes of mercury compounds into Minamata Bay. Thousands of people whose normal diet included fish from the bay unexpectedly developed symptoms of methyl mercury poisoning. The illness became known as the 'Minamata disease'. See Harada (1995). Dr Peter Hunter included details of two other environmental disasters: The Bari harbour mustard gas disaster in 1943 and the Market Drayton arsine accident of 1975. Copies of his correspondence will be deposited with the records of the meeting in Archives and Manuscripts, Wellcome Library, London.

Dayan: Which is an interesting example because the Japanese government to this day has never really admitted full responsibility for it.

Carter: The difficulties of presenting soundly-based scientific data to the public are compounded by the tendency of the media to give equal weight to an alternative view for which there is much less supporting evidence. The potential for distortion of arguments, and for increased public confusion, is obvious.

Simms: I take the point that Stanley Johnson has made about getting agreement for directives. One sometimes took the cynical view that the only way to get a directive through, or agreement for drawing up conventions at international conferences, was to agree to put the necessary restrictions in the convention on the understanding that it wouldn't be enforced. This possibly happened with the Po Valley situation. But the result of this Minamata disease, and also that with cadmium, was that the Central Unit to which Peter Corcoran and I belonged did produce what were called 'Pollution Papers', for example, summarizing the evidence of the dangers of cadmium and the dangers of mercury in the environment.[107] We didn't always get cooperation, for example, the principal polluter wouldn't give way for years on the mercury they were discharging,[108] but the cadmium experts, rather surprisingly, called a meeting and told the users to take cadmium out of the environment. They protested vigorously but surprisingly enough they did it of their own accord.

But coming back to another point about the cooperation with industry generally, I wasn't aware that the oil companies in the USA were actually cooperating on the need to prevent global warming, quite the reverse.

Dayan: When you speak of these regulatory and legislative events, and actions, they could occur in two senses or in two ways, couldn't they? One is where a problem has been fully recognized, and governments and appropriate international agreements produce the means of dealing with them, but at that stage the problem is likely to be

---

[107] Department of the Environment (1977, 1980). Dr Dennis Simms wrote: 'The Central Unit for Environmental Protection (CUEP) was formed about 1969. Initially it had an investigative function. In 1970 it was incorporated into the Department of Environment on its creation; as a sign of its importance staff were placed on the floor above that of the Secretary of State. In succeeding years, its name was changed, with "Directorate" replacing "Unit" in its title. Subsequently it moved to a different building and as reorganization followed reorganization, the name disappeared altogether while the investigative function diminished.' Letter to Mrs Lois Reynolds, 13 May 2003.

[108] On being asked for further details, Dr Dennis Simms wrote: 'I do not think the perpetrator would care to be named.' Letter to Dr Daphne Christie, 30 November 2003.

relatively serious and very well recognized. There are also examples where problems have been recognized at a much earlier stage, more as a potential than an actual problem, and action has been taken. Has there ever been any common thread historically that has led to action after the event or to action before the event, other than with intense public pressure as after Seveso and other notorious examples?

Simms: Well, that's a very difficult question to answer, but by the 1900s the Inspector of Factories was declaring that asbestos was extremely dangerous and it ought to be dealt with, and almost nothing was done.[109] I myself used asbestos in my research and in the presence of factory inspectors who knew full well the hazard they were submitting me to and they never said anything about it, so there was almost a conspiracy that some chemicals were dangerous, but nothing was done about it. Adding lead to petrol is another example of this. The US government, when it agreed to do so, relied on the evidence of Dr Kehoe in about 1926, but Dr Kehoe was also the adviser to the petrol industry. Dr Alice Hamilton who opposed putting lead into petrol was just organized out.[110]

But generally speaking, there was prescience in some cases, but nothing was done about it. The Water Pollution Research Laboratory (which was set up, I suppose, at the end of the war) had its own premises in 1952,[111] so the government was carrying out quite a lot of research into water pollution, but it took a great deal of effort before anything was done about it. Similarly the old Fuel Research Station[112] was collecting data on air pollution and what put that into effect was when all the cattle were killed in the great smog in 1952. So it takes those triggers to do it, but fortunately with the air pollution the solutions were to hand. Oil was replacing coal and so you could clean up the environment, with little extra cost; with water pollution it just required money. But by and large the old scientific principle applied, if you have got the answer when the problem arises, it's much easier to put it into effect. The trouble we found, it may have changed after I retired, that at the Directorate the problems were hitting it before we had even begun to investigate them.

---

[109] Dr Dennis Simms wrote: 'See Introduction in Bayer (1988): 5–6; although a 1902 essay by England's Inspector of Factories included the preparation and weaving of asbestos fibers as among the most injurious processes known. See also Ward (2003): 278; my last boss retired early out of frustration when she couldn't take action against a notorious large firm over asbestos dust problems from which workers are dying today, and which were well known to be dangerous then, *c*. 1955.' Letter to Dr Daphne Christie, 30 November 2003.

[110] See Graebner (1988): 15–71, in particular 41–4, 56–7 (Kehoe), 53 (Hamilton).

[111] See Melville (1962): 150–3.

[112] See Melville (1962): 153.

Hunter: In relation to the question that has just been raised – of tetraethyl lead in petrol – it was being taken pretty seriously in 1926 by Dr Joseph Aub at Harvard, who was investigating it. In fact that is when my father, Dr Donald Hunter, first became involved in industrial toxicology when he went to work for him as a research fellow in 1926.

Corcoran: I don't think we need to be too pessimistic about the ability of government to react in a precautionary manner in some cases. So perhaps this might be an opportunity to make my intervention on POPs, which stands for 'persistent organic pollutants'. The chemicals themselves, the POPs, are pretty familiar, they are the PCBs [polychlorinated biphenyls], the drins [aldrin, dieldrin, endrin], DDT and other pesticides, but also dioxins and some other chemicals, which are emitted more as by-products from incineration rather than manufactured intentionally.[113] But although those products have been largely phased out in the West, they are still extensively used in the developing world, sometimes for very good reasons like disease vector control, malaria particularly.

In the 1980s or 1990s work by one particular individual in Canada, who worked for their Native Peoples Bureau, discovered quite high levels of residues of POPs in tissue from both wild animals in the Canadian Arctic and also in people, including breast milk, at levels that were of concern.[114] I don't know whether they were showing specific effects, but they were likely to be showing more subtle effects, maybe affecting reproduction. As a result of these findings, an international convention was fairly rapidly agreed, first of all in the ECE (Economic Commission for Europe), which covers western and eastern Europe, North America and some countries like Turkey, who all agreed to phase out or reduce the use of POPs.[115] That was soon followed by a UN convention,[116] under the UN Environment Programme (the Stockholm Convention), although it was only adopted last year and hasn't yet come into effect.

---

[113] See note 115.

[114] See, for example, Hansen (1998); Hooper (1999).

[115] UN Economic Commission for Europe (UNECE). (1998) *Convention on Long-range Transboundary Air Pollution: Protocol on persistent organic pollutants.* This protocol ensured the control of the release of persistent organic pollutants – substances capable, once airborne, of being transmitted worldwide.

[116] *The UN Environment Programme: Stockholm Convention on Persistent Organic Pollutants.* (2001) The Stockholm Convention is a global treaty designed to protect human health and the environment from persistent organic pollutants. See www.pops.int/ (site accessed 2 December 2003). See also note 41.

This will put the issue of POPs on a global basis, and so eventually will involve all 180 countries within the UN, although, of course, signing up to these conventions is always voluntary. The Convention includes a financial mechanism as an added incentive to the developing countries, which requires developed countries to give technical and financial assistance to developing countries to deal with POPs. So these global issues can be addressed on an international level. It will take some time to have any effect, but the mechanism is there and, given the fact that there is a financial provision, it is likely to be effective in the longer term. Although the problems caused by these chemicals are familiar in the West, the problem of their global distribution hadn't really been addressed until these two international protocols were agreed.

Dayan: You mentioned two classes of chemicals there. One class, those substances that are deliberately manufactured because they seem to have a particular value, are tradable at a certain stage in their life cycle. The others, very often, as you said, the dioxins, arise incidentally, as a by-product of some other process, such as the incineration of rubbish, for example. The economic mechanism of the Convention that you are referring to makes it of interest to less-developed as well as to developed countries, I can see how that applies to economically valuable and profitable chemicals. How are the other substances going to be dealt with in the future? I don't think they have been dealt with at all.

Corcoran: The usual answer to that is on a case-by-case basis, which is in effect pretty much what happens. You can, for example, subsidize the disposal of waste in developing countries. I think that there is a common theme that runs through a lot of these international conventions when products and processes, which were developed in the West, are subsequently found to cause environmental problems. The developed countries used them when they were cheap and gained the benefits of doing so. As a result we have polluted large parts of the world, and now we have stopped using them and are saying to the developing world, 'Yes, well, we used them, but sorry, chaps, you can't do so because of the pollution. You must use these modern, more expensive chemicals and processes,' which are probably still only manufactured by developed countries. So, very reasonably, the developing countries say, 'The developed countries have caused this problem, and if you want us to do our bit towards preventing it becoming worse, then you must give us financial assistance to do so.'

Dayan: Very realistically, then, what you are saying is that altruism is always beaten by economics, at least at the international level.

Corcoran: Yes, but when there is an overall benefit, it's quite reasonable, I think, that there should be some transfer from the developed countries, who very often originated these problems, to the developing countries, in order too help them to avoid falling into the same trap.

Johnson: To follow Peter Corcoran's point on the international dimension of this issue, and he has mentioned POPs. I think it is also worth mentioning PIC [prior informed consent] as well, which is the convention on PIC that deals with most of the chemicals that we have been talking about and imposes certain conditions on the way in which they can be sent to other countries. For the sake of completeness – by the way, I think the PIC Convention hasn't come into force yet – one ought to add the Basel Convention on the control of these transfrontier movements of hazardous waste,[117] a very important convention. Some 135 countries have ratified it, it is in force, and developing countries are being encouraged to implement it.

There are some very extraordinary events taking place at the moment. For example, one of the things that the Basel Convention has been addressing most recently, is the break-up of ships on the coasts of Orissa in southern India, and even in Turkey, ships containing all sorts of toxic substances.[118] But I think that if we look at this whole issue of potentially toxic chemicals in the environment, it's absolutely right that one should look not just at the national, or the EU-level, mechanisms, but also these wider international conventions, and there is a move afoot now in the run-up to Johannesburg, the so-called cluster chemical conventions, to find a way in which the Basel Convention on PICs and POPs can work more effectively together.

---

[117] Mr Stanley Johnson wrote: 'The Basel Convention on the control of transboundary movements of hazardous wastes and their disposal was signed in 1989 under the aegis of the UN and came into effect on 5 May 1992. The Convention compels the signatories to ensure hazardous waste export operations are notified beforehand and exports are permitted when all parties have given their written consent. Time limits are imposed on importers for recycling and/or eliminating waste. The states undertake to refrain from transactions involving waste with countries not belonging to the Convention. In the event of imports that do not comply with the notification requirement or arriving from doubtful sources, the importing country is entitled to return the waste to the exporter.' Note on draft transcript, 12 December 2003. For more details see www.europa.eu.int/scadplus/leg/en/lvb/l28043.htm (site accessed 11 December 2003).

[118] Turkey was the first country to refuse a ship-for-scrap in 2002 on the grounds of the Basel Convention. The *Sea Beirut* containing asbestos arrived near the beaches of Aliaga and was ordered to return to France. Mr Stanley Johnson wrote: 'After 25–30 years ships are at the end of their sailing life. These "end-of-life vessels" are sold and dismantled to recover the valuable steel. About 95 per cent of the ship consists of steel. But the ships also contain large amounts of hazardous materials. Every year around 600–700 larger sea vessels are taken out of service and brought to Asia for scrap.' Note on draft transcript, 12 December 2003. For further details see www.greenpeaceweb.org/shipbreak/remarkableship_seabeirut.asp (site accessed 29 March 2004).

There is one gap, I still think, which we all need to look at. We have mentioned there are systems in the EU for evaluating both new and existing chemicals, and, of course, our EEC countries have such a system and for a time the UN was taking quite seriously something called the International Register of Potentially Toxic Chemicals (IRPTC).[119] My impression is that it is very much on the back-burner now in UN terms. So one does ask oneself if there is enough effort being made on a worldwide basis to project these protocols or whatever you want to call them in the EU and the OECD countries, on to a worldwide stage. Should we be looking for some systems whereby all people who are putting new chemicals on the market have to subject these chemicals to evaluation? I think it is worth thinking about.

Palmlund: Since we are talking about the history of environmental toxicology, I would like to raise a question that has puzzled me. As I mentioned before, in the 1960s through to the 1970s, a major environmental problem that troubled both the government of Sweden and the government of Norway were the dying lakes, crystal clear beautiful lakes with absolutely no life left.[120] The cause was what has become known as acid rain.[121] The weather patterns were very easy to interpret, it was very easy to see that much of this acid rain actually came from the UK. A number of attempts were made to ask the UK government to impose curbs on the air pollution in this country. It may be anecdotal, but I have been told that one of the first responses was to raise the height of chimneys here.[122] The problem is that that soil in southern Scandinavia is very poor in lime and you have plenty of lime here. My question is: what interest did environmental toxicologists in the UK have in this issue during the 1970s and 1980s, what sort of research was

---

[119] Mr Stanley Johnson wrote: 'The International Register of Potentially Toxic Chemicals (IRPTC) was established by UNEP in 1976, following up a recommendation of the 1972 United Nations Conference on the Human Environment held in Stockholm. The IRPTC aims to help the world community make better use of existing global resources and to give developing countries the information base to manage chemicals effectively.' Note on draft transcript, 12 December 2003.

[120] See note 42.

[121] The problem of acid rain was first observed in southern Scandinavia in the late 1950s and it was established that the origin of this pollution was in the UK and northern Europe. One early answer to industrial air pollution was to build very tall chimneys, to push polluting gases up into the atmosphere, and thus allow emissions to float away. The wind carried the pollution many hundreds of miles towards Scandinavia where it eventually fell as acid rain. The UK has contributed to at least 16 per cent of the acid deposition in Norway.

[122] The Clean Air Act of 1956, which came into effect in 1958, specified the height of chimneys. See note 136.

conducted here and what is the perspective from here over the communication with the UK government over incidences of the kind that I have mentioned?

Lovelock: I was much involved with this particular issue, and I first of all would like to ask the question, why was the UK singled out by Norway and Sweden? Perhaps I should start with an anecdote. Two of my colleagues, both Fellows of the Royal Society, were at a joint Academies meeting in Sweden on this issue, I think in the 1980s. The meeting started with the Scandinavian Chairman saying, 'Gentlemen, we are here to prove that Britain is responsible for the acid rain falling on Sweden'. I think there was an enormous degree of prejudice at the back of this story to be sure. I forget the exact figure, but I think it is about 15 per cent of the acid that fell on Sweden and Norway during that period came from power stations and other sources in the UK. But an awful lot came from other European countries, especially from eastern Europe, which at that time was exerting almost no pollution controls.

So again, I ask, why single out the UK? The factor that was left out entirely in these calculations was that a great deal of acid was coming from natural sources. The North Sea is full of algae and they produce huge quantities of dimethylsulphide that goes into the atmosphere, oxidizes to form methylsulphonic and sulphuric acids, which fall on Norway and Sweden and also on Scotland, and other places. I think the Scandinavians did have real troubles, because of the nature of the soil and the different climate there made it much more sensitive to acid rain than other parts of Europe. They did have a legitimate grievance, but I feel that their singling out the UK in this particular instance was political and not scientific.

Simms: I think Professor Lovelock has said what I was going to say, but I have one addition. It was perhaps fortunate that the days in which the westerlies blew have diminished by about 20 per cent over this period,[123] so Scandinavia got rather less than it might have done. There is a very large volume on the research that was done on this issue;[124] an awful lot of money was spent by the three governments (UK, Sweden and Norway).

Dayan: I think it would be fair to say, at least as I recall, that the early work on that form of transboundary pollution did initially suggest that with the predominantly westerly winds we might have been a major source of the acid rain that fell in Scandinavia, but subsequently, as you have said, it was realized that this

---

[123] See, for example, Holgate *et al.* (1999): 21–49.

[124] See Mason (1990).

was quite erroneous, that much of it was coming from elsewhere in eastern Europe, about which, in a sense, nothing could be done at that time, certainly not at a political level. But the memory of Britain as a major source I am afraid seems to linger in Scandinavia. We were not responsible for a lot of the problem.

Palmlund: I am quite aware that some of the sources and very important sources were in eastern Europe, but still in the 1970s the eyes were directed towards the UK. In Sweden almost every weather report that deals with low pressure in Scandinavia, starts with saying 'There is low pressure over the British Isles,' moving towards us, and so on and so forth. So everybody who listened to weather reports was very aware of the weather patterns. The meteorologists who were studying the dispersion of acid rains over southern Scandinavia were able to map out that actually there was a transport, which was not insignificant, but contributed considerably to the problem.[125] The meteorologists also, of course, were able to map the transports from the east. Since this controversy started, there has been a major research project going on concerning the transboundary air pollution in Europe, as you are probably all aware.[126]

Johnson: I think this whole question of air pollution and acid rain is very, very fascinating. Why, for example, did the EU in the mid-1980s finally agree to the air pollution emission from large industrial plant directive, which set us on the way to dealing with the question of some of these acid rain-producing emissions?[127] From my perspective, it was really what was called the 'forest die-off' in Germany, particularly at the end of the 1970s and the very beginning of the 1980s. Forests are, of course, unbelievably important to the German soul.[128] The 'die-off' moved them terrifically.

In June 1982, I think what happened at the meeting of the heads of state of the EU countries in Cologne was that the Germans finally said, 'We have had enough. We want to see a large power plant directive adopted within two years

---

[125] See note 121.

[126] See UN Economic Commission for Europe (1998). Professor Ingar Palmlund wrote: 'Research results led to further research collaboration and the creation of the Convention on Long-range Transboundary Air Pollution (see www.unece.org.env.lrtap).' Note on draft transcript, 10 February 2004.

[127] Council Directive of 28 June 1984, published in *Official Journal* L188 of 16 July 1984.

[128] Mr Stanley Johnson wrote: 'Germany was possibly the first country to recognize the loss of their woodlands in the early 1980s. In 1982 the Federal Minister of Agriculture published statistics showing that 8 per cent of the West German forests were damaged. By 1983 it had increased to 34 per cent. Since then *Waldsterben*, the German word for forest death, has became internationally known.' Note on draft transcript, 12 December 2003. See Schulze *et al.* (1989).

by the EU and Britain, and you are just going to have to come into line on this.' This is what happened.[129] Of course we were able to agree to it then, because we had some gas power plants coming on line and various others things and it was feasible for us in 1983,[130] in a way which maybe it wouldn't have been, a few years earlier. But for the purposes of this seminar, it wasn't a discrete event like an accident, but forest die-back in Germany was terrifically important to the public, and a popular event in moving air pollution policy forward.

Dayan: The second half of this afternoon will be slightly different in that we have two different areas to start us off: air pollution and water pollution. We have known something about the problems of both for a very long while, but I hope that we will hear more about them from some experts, which will lead into the more general consideration of carcinogenicity that has driven a lot of toxicology, at both the scientific level and governmental level. Certainly it has funded a lot of academic work, and has led to a great deal of activity at a governmental level, sometimes resulting in legislation. We will move on to that, and then perhaps ultimately some more general views. We have touched a little bit on the precautionary principle, but we shouldn't leave it lying doggo as it is at the moment. Please may we start on air and water pollution?

Maynard: It's important to remember that air pollution did not begin in the year of the great smog in London,[131] a period of appalling air pollution. During the first week of December 1952, perhaps 4–6000 unexpected and extra deaths occurred over those that would have been expected at that time of the year, under similar climatic conditions.[132] The event was characterized by unusually high levels of pollution in London, and the pollution in those days was due mainly to the burning of soft coal, as a means of heating houses.[133] It was a particle–sulphur dioxide mixture. The temperature was low, the air was wet and so there was a great deal of acid aerosol present as well.

Earlier we heard that some cows had died, I think, at Smithfield Market.[134] It's a great loss not to have Pat Lawther here today, because he would be able to tell

---

[129] See note 131.

[130] Mr Stanley Johnson wrote: 'Of particular importance was the shift away from coal-fired, electricity-generating plants which took place during the 1980s.' Note on draft transcript, 12 December 2003.

[131] For a history of air pollution in London see, for example, Brimblecombe (1987). See also note 136.

[132] Ministry of Health (1954).

[133] Committee on Air Pollution (1958).

[134] See page 38.

you that it was only the 'better-off' cows that died and I believe this is an important socialist point. Only the better-off cows died, because they had their bedding changed frequently, whereas the poorer-off cows, which weren't of such high quality, lived among their own ammoniacal urine which, of course, neutralized the acid in the air. So the pollution at the time was produced by capitalism and struck at capitalist animals!

This country responded to that appalling air pollution incident via the person of Sir Gerald Nabarro[135] – I don't know that he was Sir Gerald then – who was known later for his Daimler motorcars, with NAB 1, NAB 2 on the number plates, and for his fine moustache. He was the man who suggested that we should have a clean air act in this country and launched a private member's bill. There was the Beaver Committee, which had been set up to look into the problem of air pollution in London, and the private member's bill was taken over by the Government and became the Clean Air Act in 1956.[136]

It's often said that the Clean Air Act produced the enormous improvement in levels of air pollution in London and other UK cities. It played a part, but of course the increase in use of electricity and gas and oil also played a part, and so despite the fact that people were given grants for changing their heating from open coal fires into fires that would burn smokeless fuel, it's likely that air pollution levels would have been dropping by the mid-1960s. In about 1956 the MRC established the Air Pollution Research Unit, under Professor Pat Lawther's direction, at St Bartholomew's Hospital,[137] and it stayed there doing seminal work until about 1980. By then levels of air pollution had fallen to such an extent that it was beginning to be believed that not much more needed to be done. More could be done, but not much more needed to be done.

Very interestingly, it is just in the last few years that we have discovered that current levels of air pollution still have a considerable impact on health. People

---

[135] See notes 122 and 136.

[136] The Clean Air Act was passed in 1956, which aimed to control domestic sources of smoke pollution by introducing smokeless zones. See Ministry of Housing and Local Government (1956); Griffiths (1962); Berridge and Taylor (2002). See also notes 138 and 139. Further details can be found at www.pro.gov.uk/inthenews/pollution/pollution2.htm (site accessed 29 November 2003). Dr Robert Flanagan wrote: 'A further factor in the 1956 Act was that Doulton's and other Lambeth potteries that produced salt-glazed earthenware, thus liberating hydrochloric acid into the atmosphere in the firing process, lay just to the south-west of the Houses of Parliament at that time.' E-mail to Dr Daphne Christie, 29 March 2004.

[137] See biographical notes page 91.

in the audience might have heard that we calculate now that between 8000 and 10 000 deaths a year in the UK are advanced by particulate air pollution.[138] This is where the science lets us down. We know that a number of deaths have been brought forward, but we do not know by how much. So these might be very sick people whose deaths have been advanced by only a day or two and therefore perhaps are not terribly important in public health terms, but of course, the number also includes some people whose deaths have been brought forward by much longer periods, say months or years, and so that is a considerable public health impact. Until about a year ago, that was the state of play, and then a detailed reanalysis of some cohort studies undertaken in the USA has demonstrated that living for a long time, all your life if you like, in an area where levels of pollution are high, has a distinct effect on your life expectancy.[139]

I brought with me, Chairman, a book published in 1961, as this is a meeting to deal with historical aspects, and it's called *The Air We Breathe*.[140] It is the report of a symposium held in the USA. Professor Lawther was present at the symposium: he said that the role of chronic pollution in the production of disease is great, and unfortunately tends to be overshadowed by our concern with more dramatic manifestations. I think he was absolutely right. Attention has always focused on air pollution episodes, and the assumption is that between the episodes there isn't much effect on health. What we have come to understand is that it's the long-term exposure, the long-term average level of air pollution, which might be having the most significant effect on health.

This is a very worrying discovery, because if it is true, and it seems likely to be true, then it may be that there is no threshold of effect of air pollutants on health. So, Mr Chairman, the toxicology that you and I were brought up with, for example, that it must be possible for a gas like sulphur dioxide to reduce its concentration to such a level where it wouldn't have any effect – and the same goes for ozone, nitrogen dioxide, carbon monoxide and perhaps particles (although we might have known a little less about that years ago). We would have made the assumption that those common compounds would be characterized by a threshold. This may not be true and if it isn't then we can never completely solve the problem of air pollution. All we can do is to mitigate it in the UK.

---

[138] Department of Health (1998).

[139] Department of Health (2001).

[140] Farber and Wilson (1961), papers given by 31 contributors at a symposium at the University of California, San Francisco, in 1961.

Levels of particles in London are now at an all-time low. Our annual average concentration is 23 µg/m³, or thereabouts. There was a time when it was 250 µg/m³.[141] In that appalling episode in 1952, and remember this is a transient figure, not a long-term average, concentrations in London were 8000 µg/m³: averaged over about 24 hours, not a year. So we are down to 23 at the end of the twentieth century. How much further can we go? Can we reduce the level to 15 µg/m³? Yes, perhaps, but at great expense, and with difficulty. So the problem of air pollution toxicology today, not just here, but elsewhere in the world as well, is calculating the cost–benefit equation for further reductions in concentrations. What that means is that we have to move from qualitative toxicology to quantitative toxicology and as we do that, the problems of quantifying the effects of noncarcinogens and carcinogens come to the front.

For many years in the UK we have known that the air contains carcinogenic substances, and Professor Lawther referred to these in his article in 1961.[142] He said that chronic pollution and lung cancer are linked by the occurrence of substances in urban air that are known to be capable of producing experimental cancer. There is a tendency to forget that our interest in lung cancer is overwhelmingly directed to the fantastic rise in the prevalence of the disease in the last 50 years, and that's probably a result of cigarette smoking.[143] Professor Lawther was pointing out, I think, that there might be an underlying level of lung cancer, which in those days was probably more marked than now, because of the high levels of coal smoke-carrying carcinogens, but even now there may be a level of lung cancer which is attributable to air pollution. Calculating the size of that effect, or the size of the attributable risk, from air-borne carcinogens, is going to present us with a very distinct problem.

It's a problem that Professor Richard Carter and I struggled with when we were setting standards for carcinogenic air pollutants and at that time we veered fairly strongly away from attempting a quantitative risk assessment of the impact upon health.[144] As the cost–benefit equation bites, and as we come closer and closer to the limit of what we can achieve, then pressure will be put on people who know about carcinogenic mechanisms to return to that quantitative risk assessment. In the end, it will be a question of trying to explain how much more benefit you get from a very, very small reduction in a level of an air pollutant.

---

[141] See Holgate *et al.* (1999).

[142] Lawther (1961).

[143] Doll (1995); Lock *et al.* (1998).

[144] Department of the Environment (1994).

Dayan: Would anyone like to comment on any of the points that have been brought up? Or shall we bring water into the discussion as well, as there are similarities and some distinctions?

Woods: All the experts on water pollution that you invited to this meeting couldn't attend. I am, therefore, approaching this at your request in a state of aqueous innocence. The whole question of water pollution is, in my opinion, slightly different to anything else that we have been discussing this afternoon. In its historical context the major pollution of our waterways in the UK was brought to attention as a direct result of the sanitary movement in the last century, the so-called Chadwickian movement.[145] Chadwick and others in the nineteenth century pointed out the relationship between the environment and health, particularly in urban areas and to some extent in rural areas too, and the relationship between disease and waste. What happened was, of course, that the waste was put into our watercourses and rivers. So, in historical terms, this major pollution itself arose out of an effort to improve the environment.

I am a northerner, Sir, as you know, and therefore I am not going to pick on the River Thames, but I thought you might like to hear a description of the River Aire in Leeds (the town in where I was born) in 1840:

> It was full of refuse from water closets, cesspools, privies, common drains, dung hill drainings, infirmary refuse, waste from slaughter houses, chemical soap, gas, dye houses and manufacturers, coloured by blue and black dye, pig manure, old urine wash and there were dead animals, vegetable substances, and occasionally a decomposed human body.[146]

That description could have been applied to any of the rivers in the UK at that time, and what has fascinated me while reading about this is the extent to which this pollution took place. For example, at the time when a great public health advance was announced, namely the construction of sewers in London,[147] over 150 million gallons of sewage entered that river, in unit time, in one day, which

---

[145] See note 192.

[146] For further details see, for example, John Taylor Teachers Centre (n.d.).

[147] Between 1856 and 1859, 82 miles of brick-intercepting sewers were built below London's streets, all flowing by gravity, eastwards. See note 192.

was one-sixth of the total volume of the river water at that time. In other words, the proportion of the 'water' to that which was not water was extremely large.

Certain individuals had prescriptive rights to dump sewage into the Thames and that caused difficulties for legislators. Indeed, at the turn of the century, there was a great problem because those individuals insisted on their rights to continue to dump sewage into the Thames. Staines is one of the areas where they were allowed to do so.[148] The whole of the development of legislation, which is now in place in the UK, is described by those who have looked at the history of legislation in this regard, 'That it is characterized by the timidity of government in relation to bringing the legislation in', but more importantly in relation to our discussions this afternoon, 'the timidity and reluctance of government to finally decide to use the advice of experts, particularly those experts in chemistry, in order to advise them and to guide them in relation to the framing of legislation'.[149]

It wasn't until 1914 in this country that the first reasonable legislation in relation to water safety was put on the statute book in this country.[150] I don't want to labour this any further, but put this slightly in context. What are the matters that concern the consumer in this country in relation to water? We are in the fortunate position that our water supply is of very high quality irrespective of where we live in the UK. Because of this I am only going to talk about the UK. I can't remember, and I stand to be corrected, the last recorded cases of large-scale water contamination leading to bacterial illness in the UK. I am sure somebody will tell me, but it is a rare event, and we are now under legislation from the EC that governs the quality of our water.[151]

This raises another important point that I thought might be a matter for discussion, and that has been touched on this afternoon, and that is the matter of expenditure in relation to monitoring the quality of water as against the results of that checking, and whether it is economically justifiable in relation to the results.

This is somewhat heretical, particularly for somebody who chairs advisory committees – and I will tell you that I am currently chairing the third inquiry

---

[148] Wohl (1983): 233–56.

[149] See The Royal Commission on Sewage Disposal (1902–15).

[150] See note above.

[151] For UK legislation on water quality see www.ukmarinesac.org.uk/activities/waterquality/wq1_2.htm (site accessed 12 March 2004).

into the Camelford incident[152] – so I have some personal interest in this. At the moment the 1980 EC Drinking Water Directive sets a standard – and I am now talking about pesticides – of 0.1 µg/l for each pesticide.[153] I thought it would be interesting for you to know how many estimations in water under the England and Wales regulations were carried out in 2000. In the year 2000, for example, 45 000 regulatory analyses for pesticides were carried out in drinking water in England and Wales. Seven individual pesticides were detected above this level in 45 samples.[154] This means that 99.99 per cent of all samples were clear, and in every instance the concentrations found corresponded to exposures far smaller than those known to be harmful or likely to affect human health, and this raises the matter of whether once you have established a mechanism for producing a pure product, in this case water, and you have set down regulations, on how much, you should spend on its monitoring? Now that is, as I say, a somewhat heretical view, but it is one that I am interested in, because whatever we are looking at in committee somebody will say, 'Well, we should be doing more tests to see if X or Y or Z is present.'

The second point following from that is: what should we be looking for? There has been reference this afternoon to the whole business of nitrates in water and the suggestion is, as you all very well know, that levels of nitrate in water are linked in some way to the incidence of carcinoma of the stomach, there being the theoretical possibility that nitroso compounds can be generated in the stomach at certain concentrations of nitrate in humans.[155] I notice that that's all gone very quiet now, although there are still amounts of nitrate in our water. Matters move on. The final twist in this tale, which fascinates me in terms of the environment, is that having satisfied ourselves that we can turn the tap on and drink what comes out of it, we are now much more interested in what is again flowing down the rivers, and whether or not fish can live in the Thames.

[152] A third inquiry into delayed or persistent health effects of the 1988 Camelford water-poisoning incident, was set up by the Government in August 2001. The investigation followed vocal campaigning by residents who alleged that earlier inquiries did little more than 'whitewash' the incident, in which a relief driver accidentally poured 20 tonnes of aluminium sulphate into drinking water at a South-west Water treatment works. The water served people in north Cornwall. For further details see health probe into Camelford poisoning at http://news.bbc.co.uk/1/hi/uk/1490142.stm (site accessed 29 March 2004).

[153] Directive 89/778/EEC, of 15 July 1980 with its 62 measures on the 'quality of water intended for human consumption', regulates at the European pesticide level. Since 1980 the maximum admissible concentration for pesticides and related products in drinking water has been set at 0.1 µg/l per substance and at 0.5 µg/l for the sum of compounds. See Altenburger (1993).

[154] Marrs T. Personal communication.

[155] See, for example, Dupont and Cohn (1980); Pobel et al. (1995).

Dayan: You have raised a lot of issues between you, these two mass matrices that we all need. I wonder, Bob [Maynard], if you were perhaps a little unkind on the air pollution side and that there have been attempts over many hundreds of years to control it for various reasons, perhaps more aesthetic than toxicologically based, but you brought up the question of cost and benefit. Now we ought not to turn this into a seminar on political economics, but you raised serious difficulties in how you calculate the cost and benefit in the same measuring system.

Maynard: That's correct. May I say a word about the earlier history, if you like? You are quite right, of course, that there had been attempts to control levels of air pollutants, although it's fairer to say that there had been attention drawn to the undesirability of air pollution, rather than attempts made to control it. I think that's true. As you know we have [John] Evelyn's diary and also his book *Fumifugium, or, the inconvenience of the aer and smoake of London dissipated* from 1660 or thereabouts.[156] Yes, a great deal was known about it then. The Coal Smoke Abatement Society began in the 1890s,[157] the Sherlock Holmes era, the Jack the Ripper period in London, heavy smog, and that's the year or thereabouts (1903) that the word 'smog' was first coined.[158]

There was a good deal known about air pollution, but despite the fact that there were very cold winters in the late 1890s, and very high levels of pollution indeed in London, no one noticed until 1952, I think, that there were so many deaths occurring. My colleague, Robert Waller, always told me that it wouldn't have been noticed in 1952 until the coffins began to run short.[159] I don't know whether that's true or not. But it's an interesting point that if 100 more people die in London on a day would anybody notice it, as long as they were spread out across the whole city of course, and didn't all turn up in Trafalgar Square. Would you notice? The answer probably is that you would not.

---

[156] Evelyn (1661); Bray (1890).

[157] The Coal Smoke Abatement Society began in 1899. See Booth and Kershaw (1904).

[158] In 1905 Dr H A Des Voex, a member of the Coal Smoke Abatement Society in England, used the term 'smog' to describe conditions of fuliginous or sooty/smoky fogs. Smog occurs as a result of smoke particles from the domestic and industrial burning of coal becoming trapped in fog. See Wilkins (1954); Anderson (1999). See also www.vauxhallsociety.org.uk/Fog.html (site accessed 29 November 2003).

[159] Dr Dennis Simms wrote: 'The shortage of coffins was recently confirmed by a member of the Leverton family (funeral directors).' Letter to Dr Daphne Christie, 30 November 2003. See also http://news.bbc.co.uk/2/hi/health/2545747.stm (site accessed 3 March 2004).

Simms: The earliest legislation is somewhere around 1250 I think, when they tried to ban the burning of coal in London,[160] but it, like most acts, never came into effect. The first person I know who realized there was a link between air pollution and health was Roland [Rollo] Russell, who was Bertrand and Frank's uncle, although their autobiographies[161] tend to write him off as a hopeless person, but he wasn't hopeless in this direction. But nobody took any notice of him, as Professor Maynard said. Professor Maynard has rightly drawn attention to Sir Gerald Nabarro, who was, I think, funded by some of the insulation companies, but what amused me when I discussed in the Department of Environment about how the act had gone through, was that civil servants took credit for putting the act through, rather than Nabarro.[162] One of the reasons it took so long to get the act through is that Harold Macmillan didn't want it to be approved, because he didn't think it necessary.

But as I said earlier, there was the background information. The Fuel Research Station in Greenwich had collected the basic data by then. What I am concerned about, with what Professor Maynard was saying, was that it may be that the level of particulates, and the sulphur has gone down, but if you walk along most streets in London today, you will find your throat catching, because the pollution is so high. One of the things Leslie Reed wanted to do when he was in charge of this area,[163] when the oil money came on stream, was to treat ourselves to an improvement in the environment of London, but alas nothing came of it. So although the levels of old-fashioned pollutants have gone down, it seems to me that there's a very nasty cocktail developing. For example, both my grandchildren have asthma to an extent that their father never did, and I think this is a problem. It's not carcinogenicity we are bothered about, but other effects.[164]

[160] By the 1300s, the acrid smell of burning coal in London led King Edward I to ban its use. See Freese (2003).

[161] Dr Dennis Simms wrote: 'See, for example, *My Life and Adventures*, the autobiography of John Francis Stanley ('Frank'), Earl Russell (1865–1931), page 33, "…my uncle Rollo possessed the outward figure of a man…he did some good metereological work…" See also Russell (1967): 24.' Letter to Dr Daphne Christie, 30 November 2003.

[162] Dr Dennis Simms wrote: 'This remark was based on a conversation with one of them. The senior civil servant whom I challenged is still alive.' Letter to Dr Daphne Christie, 30 November 2003.

[163] See biographical note on page 92.

[164] Committee on the Medical Effects of Air Pollutants (1995); Reynolds and Tansey (2001).

Dayan: Another aspect of the curious failure to act in the area of air pollution is that of the Alkali Inspectorate,[165] which was well aware of specific problems in many areas, but took a remarkably benign view of them for a long while, didn't it?

Lovelock: Just a small point in this cost and benefit debate. It may not be well known that the sum total of air pollution in Europe, by sulphur compounds, has an appreciable climatic effect.[166] It reduces global warming quite significantly, although whether you want to call that a benefit I don't know.

Dayan: Well, a negative detriment can be a positive benefit, I suppose.

Maynard: There are several points raised by Dr Simms. On the question of the traffic-generated air pollution you are quite right, of course. In a way it has replaced the coal smoke-generated air pollution, but the levels of nitrogen dioxide that many people point to from cars, and carbon monoxide in London, are coming down at the moment and they have been coming down for a while.[167] The reason is that all new cars in the UK since 1993 have been fitted with catalytic convertors. But your point about your throat being affected, there is something in that and I don't know the answer to it, but we get complaints in the UK every summer that the air has an irritant capacity and people complain that their eyes smart and that they cough. We have had a number of possibilities raised: aldehydes (acrolein), formaldehyde. We have been round these with our advisory committees and when you measure the levels they are much lower than you would expect to produce an effect.

For what it's worth, my own guess is that fresh diesel exhaust is an irritant, and by the time you collect it and take it to the laboratory to analyse it, it's not the same as it was soon after emission from the vehicle. We know that the aerosol ages quickly and that the particle size distribution changes quickly in the air because of aggregation.

The cost–benefit analysis point is what I wanted to come to. We are now doing cost–benefit analysis on the air quality strategy for the UK, and it's

---

[165] Professor Anthony Dayan wrote: 'The Government Inspectorate established under the Alkali Act 1863 initially was to control emissions from the manufacture of hydrochloric acid and soda ash.' Note on draft transcript, 28 November 2003.

[166] Professor James Lovelock wrote: 'The effect of the aerosol haze on climate is discussed in the IPCC report [Watson (2001)]. It is thought to cool surface temperatures during the European summer by approximately 2–3°C.' Letter to Dr Daphne Christie, 9 December 2003.

[167] See Maynard and Waller (1999); Ackerman-Liebrich and Rapp (1999). See also www.defra.gov.uk/environment/statistics/airqual/ (site accessed 2 December 2003).

important not to confuse cost–benefit analysis with cost–effectiveness analysis. If you have two policies and they both produce some reduction in the number of deaths occurring per year, then you can compare them simply in terms of the number of deaths occurring per year, if you follow one policy compared with the other. But cost–benefit analysis is much more difficult and that's where you turn the health benefits into a currency that can be compared with that used to measure the costs, and as the currency used to measure the costs is invariably money, then it's important to try to turn the benefits into financial terms as well.

That means, at least in the lay mind, that you are valuing lives. We save so many lives, therefore we save so many pounds sterling and there is something repugnant about that to many people. Attempts have been made to do it using willingness-to-pay analysis,[168] and these have become more sophisticated. When I was first asked what I thought about willingness-to-pay analysis my answer was, 'Well, who are you asking me to be willing to pay for?' If it's my wife, then most days I would pay quite a lot, if it was my colleagues in the Department of Health, most days I would pay rather less. That's not how they do it, they do it in a much more sophisticated way than that, asking people how much they would be willing to pay to reduce their risks from traffic accidents or from aeroplane accidents. The Department of Transport routinely uses cost–benefit analysis to decide in the straightening of roads, dealing with bends; crashes are or were costed at about £750 000 if somebody dies. We are struggling with that in the air pollution field now. We have had a cut at it, but we haven't brought ourselves to put the benefits in monetary terms yet, but I believe we soon will have to.

Dayan: Briefly in self-defence, in a way, the cost–benefit analysis is vital, it has to come down to financial terms eventually, but as we well know from all the work that's been done by the Department of Transport and other groups in this country and elsewhere, you end up with a series of figures which become hopelessly skewed by the other factors that influence people's assessment of risk and its acceptability: £300 million per life saved for changing some minor aspect of safety in aeroplanes, opposed to about £100 000 that we are willing to spend with great reluctance on certain traffic-calming methods,[169] and ignoring the question of air pollution produced by the cars going more slowly and changing gear more often.

---

[168] Professor Robert Maynard wrote: '"Willingness-to-pay" is used as a description of a technique used by economists to estimate the monetary value people place on avoiding risk.' Note to Dr Daphne Christie, 14 November 2003.

[169] See, for example, Maddison and Pearce (1999).

Perhaps that's a bit of a side issue, but it's an intriguing one. Water seems to have managed to evade many of these cost–benefit considerations that you have brought out, Professor Woods. I don't know how or why but it has just happened. Yet again you were quoting the EU directive on drinking water with pesticide limits, which of course were set on the basis that the politicians believed that they were setting a limit of no detectable pesticide at the time when those figures were first produced. We have gone way beyond that now in the levels we can detect the pesticides but we stick to the same limits for fear of the arguments if we try to change them, I guess.

Woods: Chairman, there's another problem of course: in this seminar we are discussing air and water separately. What we have to remember, particularly in relation to pesticides, is that of course we are not singly exposed to pesticides only from water, but from a number of different sources, including food, the carpets that we walk on, the pets that we treat in the household for various infestations, and therefore it's aggregate exposure. One thing that is always forgotten with a single commodity, and the purity of that single commodity when examined, is that it is only part of a very large exposure network.

The other thing that's always forgotten is firstly that water is a very good solvent, it will also dissolve organic compounds, those of you who did any chemistry will remember that, but not to the same extent as ionic compounds. There's also a lot of it in our environment, we live in a country that has a very high rainfall. This is just an anecdote, but I was alarmed on Saturday to see a large boat in the main car park of a synagogue in a large industry city up north, and I wondered whether they knew something that I didn't in view of what is happening to the rainfall. There's also another matter that I haven't heard discussed this afternoon, that is that we are rather like dogs in this country: we like burying rubbish, and we are the largest under-the-ground buriers of rubbish, I think, in Europe. Not all of those sites are waterproof so there is potential for water to be a carrier of chemicals and other substances that are deleterious to human health, but fortunately the evidence so far in this country is that that is not a major matter.

Johnson: A number of points and questions to Professor Maynard. This morning Ken Livingstone proudly announced that second only to Athens, London now had the worst air of any major city in Europe.[170] It will be interesting to have a comment on that.

---

[170] *London Evening Standard*, 12 March 2002. For a copy of the Mayor of London's draft of the capital's first Air Quality Strategy, see www.edie.net/news/Archive/3785.html (site accessed 12 December 2003).

I have just got a couple of other things to say. One of the things I think is going to drive air pollution policy over the next decade is going to be our response to global warming as a country and as a part of a group of countries in the EC. I am quite convinced that even realizing the Kyoto commitments of an 8 per cent reduction by 2012 on 1990 levels[171] is going to produce an revolution in air pollution one way or another, because as you reduce greenhouse gases, and the HCFCs and the CFCs there will be some knock-on effects, and we have already seen it of course in the fridge mountain.[172] Why is there a fridge mountain? Because we have been not able to get rid of the freons by discarding the fridges, and so I think this is going to be quite dramatic in terms of air pollution policy. How we deal with global warming and how it will end up, whether dealing with global warming will lead to an increase in other pollutants remains to be seen, including air pollutants.

A couple of other points. If you look back over the 1960s and 1970s I think one forgets the influence of the Clean Air Society.[173] We are very used to lobby groups now like Greenpeace and Friends of the Earth, but the Clean Air Society did a rather brilliant job over a period of years pushing for legislation and achieving it, going about it in a fairly gentleman-like way.

If I could just mention a couple of things on water pollution? The intriguing thing about the current nitrate controversy, because I think it really will be a controversy, is as a result of the EU's efforts to produce a first directive dealing with nitrate load in the environment as a whole, not so much linked to the human health issue.[174] You might call it the first ecological quality standard

---

[171] The 1997 Kyoto treaty on greenhouse gas emissions requires the USA to reduce its emissions by 7 per cent below 1990 levels, the European Union by 8 per cent and Japan by 6 per cent. For further details see www.pbs.org/newshour/forum/december97/kyoto_12-12.html (site accessed 12 December 2003). See also www.unfccc.int/resource/docs/convkp/kpeng.html (site accessed 14 January 2004). Further details are provided in a note from Mr Stanley Johnson to Dr Daphne Christie, 12 December 2003.

[172] See note 98.

[173] The National Society for Clean Air was a non-governmental organization and charity founded in 1899 which campaigned for the removal of visible smoke, particularly from coal, from the urban landscape. Mr Stanley Johnson wrote: 'Now renamed as the National Society for Clean Air and Environmental Protection (NSCA), with the objectives of promoting clean air through the reduction of air, water and land pollution, noise and other contaminants, while having due regard for other aspects of the environment. It examines questions of environmental policy from an air quality perspective and aims to place them in a broader social and economic context. It organizes conferences, workshops and seminars, and publishes a journal.' Note on draft transcript, 12 December 2003.

[174] See Council Directive of 12 December 1991 concerning the protection of waters against pollution caused by nitrates from agricultural sources.

directive we have had. Of course part of that was stimulated by the situation in Holland where you have so many pigs per square metre, you can practically smell the pollution on the east coast of the UK coming over the Channel, so I think that's going to be a really intriguing debate.

Another question to Frank Woods: is it absolutely too late, in investment terms, to reverse this idea of putting all our solid wastes into the water? It has always struck me as being a most extraordinary idea that we do it, but is it possible to imagine going back to a pre-Chadwick system here? Are we condemned to have a situation where sewage and drinking water are always combined?

Woods: I hope sewage and drinking water aren't always combined. It's an interesting point. I must stress that I am not an expert in this area, but as an observer of this, we do do some work on chemical contamination of water. The whole matter of how we deal with sewage in this country has become a matter of aesthetics, not necessarily a matter primarily driven by public health. It relates, of course, to the beaches and the sea around the coast, and there is continual pressure leading to substantial expenditure on further treatment of sewage, rather than dumping it raw into the oceans. That, of course, is the last aspect of this, because what we put into our rivers – and we still put quite a lot of inorganic and organic compounds into our rivers – ends up in the sea. We are a country that does depend on the sea for part of our food, and therefore it enters the food chain, in fish which themselves concentrate certain of these chemicals, both inorganic and organic, so it is a very complex chain.

Farmer: Just a quick point. From a toxicological point of view I think this debate emphasizes how important it is that we know more about the dose–response relationship at these low doses of exposure, because if you don't know what happens you are not then going to be able to calculate the positive health effect of the effort involved in reducing exposure levels. Over the last 30 years or so, I think there have been dramatic advances for some types of compounds like genotoxic carcinogens,[175] but the situation for biomarkers for nongenotoxic carcinogens is not nearly so clear and in this case of course we are saying that there may well be a threshold of that exposure where there's no risk. I just wanted to emphasize that I think it's really important that we keep the research side going for the study of these low dose–response relationships.

---

[175] Professor Peter Farmer wrote: 'The initiation stage of carcinogenesis for genotoxic carcinogens is believed to be the interaction of the compound with DNA. For genotoxic carcinogens it is normally assumed that there is no discernible threshold and any level of exposure carries some degree of carcinogenic risk.' Note on draft transcript, 24 November 2003.

Maynard: Chairman, a number of points. I am too old a dog to be drawn on the question of whether London is the second worst city in Europe. It depends, I guess, on what figures are used in terms of averaging times, because that's usually the problem with these comparisons. Athens and all southern European cities have very high ozone levels and that's simply due to sunlight. They also have high particle levels, and that's due to diesel vehicles on the whole. I am not sure whether we are second to the others. You also raised a point about global warming, and that is an important point certainly, and so is our policy on waste disposal, which you touched on in the discussion going back to a pre-Chadwick approach. As I understood this, it was that you chucked waste in the street and walked on it. *Gardez l'eau*, Chairman, and that wasn't what you meant, of course. We want a better solution than chucking it in the street.

The new European directive on waste disposal[176] is going to force us down the incineration route and away from land fill, and that means that the problem of waste disposal will become mine, because incinerators cause air pollution, and not Frank's, where waste burial might cause water pollution. Thank you for the problem! The real difficulty is that we are in at low levels, and it's Peter Farmer's point about the effects at these levels and therefore can the benefits be calculated? Our recent evidence is all based on one sort of epidemiological study.[177] We do not know the toxicological mechanisms by which low levels of ozone, particles, sulphur dioxide, nitrogen dioxide or carbon monoxide actually affect health. All standard toxicology would say that at the levels we see today there would be no effect on health, and yet the modern epidemiological techniques reveal effects at these levels and allow us to draw dose–response curves. We are in grave difficulties, and we certainly do need more research on it. The question of whether the country has the capacity to pay for the level of safety that is currently desired, or is asserted to be desired by some people, I think is a terribly important and very deep question. I am beginning to think that it is not sustainable. The cost will become extremely high and will be difficult to maintain from public resources.

I am reminded of an anecdote I heard from Mr Sidney Weighell, who some people here will remember was in charge of the Railway Workers' Union at the time [1975]. His father had been a railwayman as was his grandfather before him. On retirement he was asked some questions on television and commented on the state of the railways (and this is not an exact quotation, so I wouldn't want

---

[176] See, for example, www.europa.eu.int/comm/environment/waste/index.htm (site accessed 2 December 2003).

[177] See Samet and Jaakkola (1999).

to be held to account for it) but I think his point was that you cannot run the sort of railway that most people would like without a very large, very underpaid workforce, and that's exactly what we had in this country, when we had the sort of railway that all middle-class people liked. They could look up in their *Bradshaw*[178] when the train would be leaving King's Cross for Edinburgh, there were fires in the waiting rooms, there were men to carry your bag to the train, somebody to give you a rug and to hand in the hamper. If you had to pay for that now at a reasonable rate, you would choose not to pay for it, and would board the train under your own steam.

Lovelock: I was prompted to comment on the Ken Livingstone remark, comparing London and Athens. I think it's much more sensible to look at most of Europe as one large city. I have measured air pollution even in places such as far-western Ireland. Ozone there can be way above the EPA safety limits – 100 parts per billion of ozone is not unusual.[179] Air pollution is everywhere, all over Europe and singling out cities is not really wise. The other point is about sewage. In my experience living in a rural area, the output of sewage from farms – cattle effluent – so exceeds anything human that it's almost ridiculous to fret about what people are doing, when one considers what farmers are doing with their cattle, and the practice of slurry farming, where you have more cattle than you would normally put on a piece of land and you use the piece of land as a disposal site for their effluent, is dreadful, especially in a country with increasing rainfall. It all goes into rivers. The fish in the river where I live have all died long ago, and oxygen levels go down to zero in wintertime. This used not to be the case when farmers put nitrates on the field.

Dayan: It is intriguing and I don't know how it can readily be dealt with, but air pollution, as you say, has to be dealt with on at least a continental level, the political unit has to be enormous. Water for the moment, at least in this country, is one of the benefits of being an island, isn't it? We can deal with it on a national basis perhaps, although I don't know how long that will continue either.

Simms: First of all, I have remembered the one incident of water being polluted by sewage that occurred in my time. A group of doctors used to dine together in, I think, Yorkshire. They noticed an increase in cases of diarrhoea and informed the local water board. It was discovered that the farmers' sewage was going past four

---

[178] *Bradshaw's Guide* is a detailed, national, UK railway timetable, first published 1839, in print until 1939.

[179] The Environmental Protection Agency (EPA)'s National Ambient Air Quality Standard for ozone is a maximum eight-hour average outdoor concentration of 0.08 parts per million (or 80 parts per billion). See Cox *et al.* (1975).

wells and the sampling that the local water authority had devised meant that only three of the wells were tested. I don't know quite how this happened, but the sewage was running into the fourth well, which was the one that wasn't being tested. That was the only case I remember being brought to headquarters in about 15 years, but that was tummy ache only. I think I have to disagree with you, Chairman, about water pollution and isolation. There are a number of international conventions that control what we can let out of our estuaries and rivers. Firstly there are the Oslo and Paris Conventions, now called the OSPAR Convention,[180] which severely limits what you can discharge; the London Dumping Convention,[181] which is global and a subject that hasn't been raised very much today; there was the IMO [International Maritime Organization] Convention, I think it was in 1974, that dealt with oil pollution.[182] So there is a whole series of conventions, which grew out of the Stockholm conference in the early 1970s. There are also obligations under the third UN Law of the Sea Convention.[183] We can't discharge what we like, but what we do discharge, there is control in that respect at any rate.

Dayan: Sorry. Inadvertently I gave the wrong impression – it's a long while since we suffered from the foaming rivers due to the inappropriate detergents.

Corcoran: I am going to adopt the rather unpopular position of defending farmers. I think they have been getting a fair amount of stick in this meeting. Agriculture is not the only source of pollution even by pesticides. Large quantities of pesticides are used for nonagricultural purposes, often by local authorities on parks, gardens and particularly roads, and whoever owns the railways nowadays uses a fair amount to control weeds on rail tracks. So quite a lot of the pollution, particularly of surface and ground water, has come from

---

[180] Dr Dennis Simms wrote: 'The OSPAR Convention is the combination of the Oslo Convention, which has the same objectives as the London Dumping Convention, and the Paris Convention (see note 196).' Letter to Dr Daphne Christie, 19 February 2004.

[181] The London Dumping Convention (Convention on the Prevention of Marine Pollution by Dumping of Wastes and Other Matters), 1972, was established to control pollution of the sea by dumping of wastes that could create hazards to human health or harm living resources and marine life, damage amenities, and interfere with other legitimate uses of the sea. See also www.imo.org/Conventions/ and www.unep.ch/seas/main/legal/llondon.html (sites accessed 4 May 2004). International Maritime Organization (1991).

[182] International Convention relating to Intervention on the High Seas in Cases of Oil Pollution Casualties (Intervention), 1969 (1975); Protocol of 1973 (1983).

[183] For an overview and full text of the United Nations Convention on the Law of the Sea of 10 December 1982 see www.un.org/Depts/los/convention_agreements/convention_overview_convention.htm (site accessed 12 December 2003).

nonagricultural use of pesticides.[184] Contracts often specify that no weeds must appear within a specified period, such as nine months, so there has been an incentive to use large quantities of herbicides. We must remember that there are other sources of pesticide pollution than agriculture. Recently, of course, the whole of farming has been under scrutiny following BSE and foot and mouth disease.[185] This includes the recent Curry Report,[186] which suggested that the whole emphasis of farming policy should swing away from intensive food production towards protection of the environment, resulting in reduced use of pesticides and fertilizers, and perhaps more land going to set-aside or being used as wildlife reserves. So there are overarching policy moves away from some practices that have caused pollution in the past.

Dayan: Going back to the Oslo and the Paris Conventions in the mid-1970s both affected to a great extent what was released into water. But what led to those conventions – why did countries accept those constraints?

Simms: I wasn't directly concerned with the origins of the Oslo or Paris Conventions, but I was concerned with the London Dumping Convention and the Marine Pollution Convention,[187] in as far as I can make out there was a general worry that the seas were becoming polluted. Peter Walker, who was the Minister of the Environment at the time, made an offer at Stockholm to hold a meeting on dumping in London. Behind all this there was the UN Third Law of the Sea Conference[188] and that too had had a section on the prevention of marine pollution. That was due to a Maltese professor whose name now escapes me, who made a long speech at the UN on the dangers to the marine world and as a result the conference was set up. The Baltic Convention was the result of the Scandinavians getting extremely angry at the amount of untreated sewage washing up on their shores from Leningrad, as it was then. There was also a Mediterranean Convention on the Prevention of Marine Pollution that was set up, because, as I

---

[184] Department of the Environment, Central Unit on Environmental Pollution (1974).

[185] See Reynolds and Tansey (2003).

[186] The Policy Commission on the Future of Farming and Food was established in 2001 to advise the Government on how to create a sustainable, competitive and diverse farming and food sector, chaired by Sir Donald Curry. See Policy Commission on the Future of Farming and Food (2002). For further details see www.epolitix.com/data/companies/images/Companies/Countryside-Agency/Curry.htm (site accessed 2 December 2003). For the full terms of reference of the Policy Commission see www.defra.gov.uk/farm/sustain (site accessed 3 March 2004).

[187] See note 181.

[188] See note 183.

say, people were just becoming concerned. If you like it was just a *zeitgeist* as far as I could make out and I wasn't happy with it, I was being kept too busy!

Hunter: I would just like to say something about the survival of patients with chronic lung disease during fogs and smogs. In the late 1950s and early 1960s during heavy fogs and smogs, it was not unusual for there to be 20 or more patients with respiratory failure on trolleys in corridors of the Central Middlesex Hospital in north-west London.[189] The majority were chronic bronchitics many of whom had chronic CO_2 retention. Quite a few of these patients would have been killed by the administration of unrestricted oxygen. That they survived was largely due to the work of a single man: Dr Moran Campbell. He studied the effects of chronic CO_2 retention, which led to the development of the Venturi mask,[190] which delivers precisely graduated percentages of oxygen in to the patient's inspired air. He subsequently became the first Professor of Medicine at McMaster University in Kingston, Ontario, Canada.

If I can briefly go back to what was said about the development of knowledge about how dangerous polluted water was. An absolutely key figure in that area was the medical statistician, Dr William Farr, who published a study in which he measured mortality from water-borne disease in London according to the altitude above the Thames,[191] in about 1850. This was one of the things that stirred Sir Edwin Chadwick, whose great by-word was 'circulation not stagnation', and he got together with a very, very remarkable man, Joseph Bazalgette, who constructed the main sewage system of London.[192] I don't know if any of you have ever seen a map of that, but at least two of these sewers are actually longer than some of the longer London Underground lines.

Maynard: I was just going to contrast the position in the air pollution field with the position in the water field at the moment. In the air pollution field we have new epidemiological methods, which has allowed us to detect effects of very, very low concentrations. Effects that in toxicological terms we can't understand. But

---

[189] Dr Peter Hunter wrote: 'I did a three-month clinical attachment there as a student during my clinical years at the Middlesex Hospital, between 1960 and 1963. The Clean Air Act of 1956 gave powers to the Alkali Inspectorate to ensure that the best practicable means of prevention of emissions "of dark smoke, grit or harmful gases", were put into operation. These new responsibilities extended the Alkali Acts to cover 11 more classes of works, with effect from 1 June 1958 [see Hunter D (1978): 151–2].' Note to Dr Daphne Christie, 25 November 2003.

[190] See the Glossary, page 97.

[191] See Farr (1856): 74–99.

[192] Chadwick (1842); Bazalgette (1864–5). See also Farr (1867–8); Halliday (2001).

in the water field it seems to me that you have measurements of very, very low levels of compounds that are known to be toxic, but you don't have methods to detect whether effects are occurring in the population. I wonder why that is? Why has the air pollution field been particularly favoured (if that's the word) with this epidemiological advance?

Woods: I don't want to rise to that point. It's not just water, Bob [Maynard], as you know. We are hampered in relation to chemical toxicity, as we alluded to earlier this afternoon, by the lack of markers of effect. We are also hampered to some extent – and there's a report coming out very shortly on this subject[193] – by the methodology for aggregating the exposure from various sources for a common set of compounds, for example pesticides. We are very good at concentrating on pesticides in water or in food, but what we are not so good at is aggregating these effects across the whole of the human exposure. To Dr Hunter: if you look at the January edition of *Medical History*[194] you will see a very good paper in relation to Chadwick and the statistics that you mention, and the whole criticism of Chadwick's approach to living. I can't remember his exact terminology now, but there was criticism of the way in which he used statistics, and the way he derived a measure of human survival.[195]

Johnson: I wish I was Doctor. As just Mister, I feel very humble in this illustrious audience. Taking a historical perspective on the water pollution side, I think it is quite interesting to see how much we do owe to the Paris Convention. I was present in early 1974 at most of the negotiating sessions of the Paris Convention,[196] which, surprisingly enough, took place at the Centre Kleber. The object of that convention was and is to control land-based pollution, what the French call *pollution tellurique*.[197] The annexes of the Convention document contain the usual suspects in terms of the well-known chemicals and they are more or less the same on any list of chemicals you wish to control. I think the

---

[193] A report of the Committee on Toxicity (COT) in 2003 on multiple pesticide exposure. See www.foodstandards.gov.uk/science/research/chemsafety/t10prog/?version=1 (site accessed 10 March 2004).

[194] Hanley (2002).

[195] Chadwick (1842). Chadwick's chosen statistical measure – the average age at which a given class of people died – was calculated by adding up the ages of all who died and dividing the total by the number of deaths.

[196] See note 180. The Convention for the Prevention of Marine Pollution from Land-based Sources (the 'Paris Convention') was opened for signature in June 1974 and entered into force in 1978.

[197] Pollution of marine waters from land-based sources.

annexes are pretty the much the same as Oslo, for example, barring, I think, the question of radioactive waste.

But what I wanted to get at was the impact of the Paris Convention on the evolution of EU water pollution policy. As a direct result of the Paris Convention and of the fact that there was at exactly that time a draft convention on the pollution of the Rhine in the offing, which was worked out within the framework of the Council of Europe (not to be confused with the European Council).[198] Precisely because of that the EU came forward in 1976 with its first directive on the control of the quality of dangerous substances discharged into water. It was known as the famous ENV 131 and the adoption of that directive in May 1976[199] set the scene for the further antipollution policy.

But what was very significant was the very hard-fought battle by the British, and it was a Labour government who were then in power, because we are talking about 1976 with Dennis Howell[200] in the lead, as junior minister to Peter Shore.[201] They said,

> Look, we do not believe the way to control the presence of toxic chemicals in the environment is through emission standards. We believe the way to do it is through the setting of quality objectives, and we want to have that opportunity and that possibility or proceed on that basis. We do not want to be told that we have to impose certain emission standards on our industries.[202]

They fought and they fought, and finally the upshot was that a dual approach was agreed. Finally, there has been a recognition in the last few years that both

---

[198] Mr Stanley Johnson wrote: 'The Council of Europe is the continent's oldest political organization, founded in 1949. It groups together 45 countries, including 21 from central and eastern Europe. It is distinct from the 15 (soon to be 25) nations in the European Union (which has its own Council), but no country has ever joined the Union without first belonging to the Council of Europe.' Note on draft transcript, 12 December 2003.

[199] Mr Stanley Johnson wrote: 'ENV 131 was the symbol under which the draft directive was discussed in 1975 and 1976 in the Environment Working Group of the Council. Adopted on 4 May 1976 (OJ No. L129 of 18/5/1976) its full title was "The directive on pollution caused by certain dangerous substances discharged into the aquatic environment".' Note on draft transcript, 12 December 2003.

[200] Mr Dennis (later Lord) Howell.

[201] Secretary of State for the Environment from 1969 to 1979.

[202] Mr Stanley Johnson wrote: 'UK Ministers of the time tended to believe that Britain's short fast-flowing rivers and turbulent surrounding seas gave British industry a competitive advantage as far as the disposal of effluent was concerned, an advantage which could be negated or diminished by the imposition of uniform emission standards.' Note on draft transcript, 12 December 2003.

policies are probably needed – the quality objective policy and the emissions standards policy – and what we now have about to be implemented within the EU is the new water framework directive[203] which is going to go down both routes. There will be quality standards set for the receiving environment but also emissions standards set for the major discharges of these key pollutants.

Smith: Could I just attempt to rise to the bait from Professor Maynard? He was citing pieces of evidence, which would be music to a particular group of advocates: the clinical ecologists. They believe in multiple chemical sensitivity, and believe that there are a number of human syndromes that have no counterpart, certainly in terms of animal toxicology, and above all that there are no dose–response curves available. I wonder if he was mildly beginning to propose multiple chemical sensitivity as being an acceptable condition?

Maynard: No. The longer answer is that the epidemiological studies are sound, fascinating, and difficult to understand, but we now have a database that the Department of Health pays for, of more than 150 epidemiological studies looking at day-to-day changes in levels of particles, for example. Although the statistics are complex, they have been crawled over in such detail by industry who were dumbstruck by the results, but I believe there is nothing wrong with the statistics and our statistical advisers agree. I think the relationship is there and we are struggling with the mechanism.

But just recently something has turned up, which I don't think anybody in the air pollution field would have expected, and that is data from monitoring people's heart rate. These are records from people who have been wearing monitors because they either have in-dwelling pacemakers or are being monitored to see if they need a pacemaker. Analyses of these records have shown that heart-rate variability tracks with the small changes in air pollution.[204] That's not just whether it's 60 a minute or 50 a minute or 70 a minute, it's the beat-to-beat variability, so that your heart rate at the moment might be 70 a minute and so might mine, but my heart-rate variability might be more than yours, the gaps might be more variable between my individual beats, despite the fact that we

[203] On 23 October 2000, the 'Directive 2000/60/EC of the European Parliament and of the Council establishing a framework for the Community action in the field of water policy' (or the EU Water Framework Directive) was finally adopted. Details can be found at www.europa.eu.int/comm/environment/water/water-framework/index_en.html (site accessed 12 March 2004).

[204] Magari *et al.* (2002).

have the same heart pulse rate. The funniest thing of all is that it's the cardiovascular effects that are more important than the respiratory effects.

I felt exactly as you do about ten years ago when this stuff started to come out, that nobody would believe it at this low level. It has been fascinating to see the way in which committee opinion has changed. The committee that I look after is the Committee on the Medical Effects of Air Pollutants. I remember the early meetings, Professor Dayan, I think you were there, when people were saying, 'These levels are so low in comparison with levels that we regard as safe in occupational conditions, so how could there possibly be an effect on health? How could that possibly work?' But though I take your point, I am anxious that we don't stray across the line into difficulties like multiple-chemical sensitivity.

Dayan: At least in terms of conditions you mentioned you are dealing with well-defined entities that can be subjected to quite vigorous epidemiological analysis, as opposed to what the clinical ecologists are usually bombarding us with.

Sir Christopher Booth: I speak as a clinician of some years standing and my only connection with the toxicology field is having chaired the British Medical Association's Board of Science's report on pesticides some years ago.[205] What I can recall is how very low the concentrations were that people were trying to persuade us to be concerned about. So far as the clinical world is concerned, I have to say that the concept of clinical ecology does not have tremendous support among working-class clinicians, if I might put it that way. One of the reasons for this is because the individuals who practise it are in business in Harley Street to demonstrate that somebody has an allergy to some strange thing that they say they have an allergy to. In my opinion, most of what they do is baloney.

Dayan: Perhaps we had better leave that point rather hastily. Coming back to both water and air pollution, one of the very many interesting things that has been mentioned is that one has become accustomed to doing various sorts of laboratory tests in an attempt to predict potential harm, dose–response relationships and so on. One of the areas that has attracted a lot of attention, as with the pesticides we discussed earlier, is carcinogenicity. The notion has been to try to set a tolerable limit on a carcinogen, whatever it may be, to which we are perhaps exposed inescapably every day, by taking some sort of animal data, and possibly some sort of epidemiological data, and extrapolating it a long long way, down to, say, air or water pollution levels. It's done and perhaps demonstrably done effectively, but it's worrying in other ways. Professor Carter, you have had long experience of this magic art.

---

[205] British Medical Association (1990).

Carter: Before I deal with your question I would like to make a few more general comments. Rachel Carson taught us that pre-existing environmental toxins, irrespective of their nature and effects, can be increased by casual human activity; and above all that many new toxins can be easily introduced, impinging on sparsely populated areas of intensive agriculture as well as on regions of urban development. To assume that the original natural environment in such circumstances was pristine is not really sustainable, and you may feel that the term 'natural environment' is in any case a rather loose one. I am using it here because it does provide a contrast to the occupational environment – the essentially contrived setting in which a small and selected workforce may encounter toxins under unusual conditions with respect to amount, route and duration of exposure. When *Silent Spring* was published 40 years ago, environmental carcinogens would, I think, have been sought primarily in industrial and occupational settings.[206] Today the field is wider and more diffuse, and I see the issue more as carcinogenic hazards and risks among broadly-based populations, living in natural environments, which are being changed (usually irreversibly) as a consequence of economic development.

I would like to make four points. First, to remind you that underdeveloped natural environments are not carcinogen-free. Consider aflatoxin B1 in stored cereals contaminated by *Aspergillus flavus*, or arsenic salts occurring in certain waters from natural sources.[207] Oesophageal cancer in Iran (a high-incidence area) is probably due to a dietary carcinogen, but three features are worth noting about this condition.[208] It is concentrated in the southern part of the Caspian Littoral; it is ancient with plausible descriptions dating back several hundred years; and it occurs mainly among people who have retained their traditional lifestyle. Secondly, the sorts of carcinogens that may impinge on people living in developing natural environments will obviously vary. Some familiar carcinogens may persist, some may recur, and new carcinogens, possibly whole new classes, may be described in the future. But the context in which they will probably operate is important. Thus, exposure is likely to be more often to mixtures than

---

[206] Dr Dennis Simms wrote: 'The first modern writer to provide detailed accounts on the effects of pollutants on the workman was Bernadino Ramazzini (1633–1714) in 1700. An English edition appeared in 1705 titled *The Diseases of Workmen*.' Letter to Dr Daphne Christie, 30 November 2003. See Ramazzini (1700, 1705).

[207] See International Agency for Research on Cancer (1980, 1993).

[208] See Mahboubi *et al.* (1973). Professor Richard Carter wrote: 'These observations are of great interest and it is hoped that, given greater political stability in the region, the work can be developed further.' Note on draft transcript, 1 December 2003.

to pure carcinogens and it will tend to involve low doses over long periods, perhaps most or all of a lifetime. Environmental and lifestyle carcinogens, notably tobacco, may interact. The target population will be diverse in almost all respects, unlike a workforce. That is, both sexes, all ages (perhaps with an age-related susceptibility) and different occupations, lifestyle and mobility.

Thirdly, there seems to be something of a change over the last 40 years in the way that carcinogenic risks from the environment (actual or putative) are perceived and formulated. There is rather less emphasis on a specific carcinogen and its congeners, and greater emphasis on what you might call more general carcinogenic risks which are often difficult to evaluate. For instance, the effects of ambient air pollution from fixed sources and from vehicle exhausts, which Bob [Maynard] was talking about, or dietary factors.

Lastly, some putative carcinogens may be close to or beyond the limits of currently available methods of investigation, that is in terms of conventional epidemiology or conventional toxicology. Additional approaches are needed. Since *Silent Spring* there have, of course, been major advances in our understanding of carcinogenesis. Consider the distinctions we were talking about earlier between genotoxic and nongenotoxic mechanisms, the increasing range of molecular investigations (linking with aetiology) that can be done directly with *human* tissues, and the emergence of molecular epidemiology in areas such as biomarkers.[209] Even more sensitive analytical methods for detecting minute amounts of toxic chemicals are increasingly available, although they raise important problems in evaluation that are more appropriately discussed by Peter Farmer. Encouraging though these various developments may be, it would be deplorable if Rachel Carson's work was regarded as obsolete and be forgotten.

Dayan: Would you care to add anything specifically about carcinogenicity and testing for it, or perhaps you have said it all?

Carter: Testing for putative carcinogens has improved to the extent that we can now separate them into two operational groups. For genotoxic carcinogens we have acceptable short-term testing procedures and prediction in terms of chemical structure for the parent compound or for its metabolites.[210] This information should reduce the need for long-term carcinogenicity testing when dealing with such compounds. Nongenotoxic carcinogens present major problems because there are no standard short-term predictive tests and no guides are provided by

---

[209] Miller *et al.* (2001).

[210] McGregor *et al.* (1999).

the chemical structure of the suspected compounds. Their underlying mechanisms of action are diverse and for the most part poorly understood. You also have the problem of marked species variation in response to nongenotoxic carcinogens. Several compounds are known to induce tumours in one sex or one strain of one species and are of no relevance to humans. The urgent need is to clarify the basic mechanisms of nongenotoxic carcinogens especially, as I said earlier, because many human carcinogens are likely to fall into this category.

Maynard: Richard, could we turn to another point, perhaps? You and I have often discussed the difficulties of quantitative risk assessment for carcinogens, and many countries use a system whereby they predict the impact of exposure to a carcinogen at an environmental level of exposure, and they do that by extrapolating either from data obtained in animal experimentation (and that perhaps is the least satisfactory) or sometimes from data obtained in occupational epidemiological studies. So we have a series of problems: we have the problem of species extrapolation and we have the problem of extrapolation from high doses where effects are comparatively obvious to low doses where effects certainly are not obvious at all and how to make that extrapolation using some sort of model. You and I have agreed over the years that current practice is not likely to produce a reliable answer or perhaps more importantly, an answer that can be tested against the facts. I wonder whether you think the field is improving, or not, or whether we are stymied. I guess you may think it hasn't improved a great deal since you and I last spoke about it, but if we are stymied, what research do we need to help us go forward with that? Is it in the biomarker area? Is that what we should be attacking?

Carter: As Bob has said, we have the problems of extrapolating data first *within* one species from high-dose levels to low-dose levels, the shape of the curve towards the lower end being little known or indeed not known at all; and then *across* species from test animals to humans. Secondly there are difficulties in choosing the most appropriate biomathematical models on which to base quantitative risk assessment for a human population. Even if you use only human-based data, for example the incidence of leukaemias (particularly acute myeloid) in workers exposed to benzene,[211] different models will yield different answers in terms of putative risk. Recent models have, however, more biological and, in particular, toxicokinetic plausibility, and may provide results with greater predictive value which are applicable in environmental as well as industrial and occupational contexts.

---

[211] Professor Richard Carter wrote: 'The literature on the leukaemogenic effects of benzene in humans is large, but a useful summary may be found in Department of the Environment (1994).' Note on draft transcript, 1 December 2003.

Farmer: I agree with absolutely everything that Professor Carter has just said and this problem of high- to low-dose extrapolation, especially between animals and man, still does exist. Another problem is that the high-dose exposures are normally associated with occupational exposure, which is often to a single or a very small number of chemicals, and the low-dose exposures are normally associated with very mixed exposures, such as in environmental pollution. For example, for benzene, occupational exposure involves benzene as a major component, but environmental pollution with benzene is associated with very complex mixtures and particles and so on. I think the way to look forward is probably, as has been indicated, with biomarkers. The people working in genotoxic carcinogenesis are getting much better now at identifying molecular interactions of these compounds with DNA, which leads to the possibility of predicting specific mutational effects, which again leads to the possibility of predicting some type of carcinogenic risk from it. The sensitivity of these methods is such that they can cope with this large dose range between the occupational and the environmental exposure.[212] So we are not there yet, but I think we are on the way to establishing some sort of dose–response relationship over these different types of exposure.

Lovelock: On the matter of setting safe levels for carcinogens, it comes to my mind that natural carcinogens such as ultraviolet radiation have benefits as well as demerits, and setting a level is going to be quite a tricky problem. Perhaps the most extreme example is oxygen itself, which one could argue quite strongly is the ultimate carcinogen. One obviously cannot ban it. [**From the floor:** We could tax it.]

Smith: I think that one of the problems that we face here is that our present-day testing methods give you estimates of hazard, but not of risk. I think the UK public ought to be reassured that our testing methods for carcinogens and probably reproductive toxins have been pretty good for the past 30 or 40 years. I can think of very few examples where a major carcinogen, a human carcinogen, or reproductive toxin, has got into the human exposure chain. The problem for me is a number of regulatory organizations now seem to respond to the hazard. For example, and I can give you a current one, the German government have just banned the use of methyl eugenol, which is the main component of basil (for those who like pesto). They banned it on the basis of an NTP study where the lowest-dose level was about 10 000 times that of human exposure. Another example of the undue haste of regulatory bodies to respond to hazard estimates

---

[212] See Hemminki *et al.* (1994); Toniolo *et al.* (1997).

is California Proposition 65; they are about to ban the use of coumarin.[213] This is our problem now, the crazy move from hazard estimate to the precautionary principle of banning these materials, and I think many innocent compounds are being damaged through this process, Chairman.

Dayan: It would be quite interesting, but we haven't the time now to go round to each of you and ask you to define what you mean by the precautionary principle. It's a somewhat elastic entity these days, isn't it, or an elastic notion? Professor Lovelock, do you wish to say something in general at this stage, in relation particularly to the precautionary principle?

Lovelock: Thanks to Rachel Carson we are aware of the harm we can do to the natural environment, but in spite of her warnings, things have got a lot worse for wildlife. There is almost a *Silent Spring*, but it's not simply due to pesticide poisoning, but rather to the widespread loss of habitats as population and energy consumption has increased. According to E O Wilson, who is a most eminent biologist, it would take five earths to provide food and resources needed to sustain the present world population at US standards of living.[214] I don't know how much that exaggerates the position. I do know that it has been estimated that even now we are using more than 60 per cent of the photosynthetic capacity entirely for our own needs. Does it matter? Why couldn't we farm the entire land surface and take from the ocean its maximum sustainable output. I think we can't do it, because we need the earth's natural habitats to sustain the favourable climate and chemistry that we now enjoy. There is little reason to believe that the monocultures of farmland would fill this role as well as do the evolved natural habitats.

In spite of the splendid science of the Intergovernmental Panel on Climate Change (IPCC)[215] and other scientific groupings, we still know far too little

---

[213] Proposition 65, passed into law in 1986, was created to improve public health through the reduction of the incidence of cancer and adverse reproductive outcomes that might result from exposure to potentially hazardous chemicals, by restricting discharges of listed chemicals into known drinking water sources. A clear and reasonable warning must be given under the Act prior to a known and intentional exposure to a listed substance.

[214] Wilson (2002). See also Lovelock (1971).

[215] The Intergovernmental Panel on Climate Change (IPCC) was created by the WMO and UNEP in 1988, as the scientific research arm of international efforts to control climate change. The Panel includes climatologists, scientists and government officials from more than 100 nations, and is divided into three working groups: one to review and assess the causes of climate change; a second to assess the possible environmental and socioeconomic impacts of climate change; and a third to identify potential response strategies. See Watson (2001).

about the earth system to be able to make useful predictions. We are just now passing through one of the brief interglacial periods of warmth in the earth's history, between the long periods of the ice ages. From the systems viewpoint, an interglacial is like a fever in a mammal: it's a state dominated by positive feedback, so that the effects of greenhouse gases and habitat removal are amplified not resisted, and this is reflected in the wide range of predicted consequences of global warming as the century proceeds: 6°C at the worst, and 2°C for the more optimistic forecast.[216] I would add that even a two-degree rise has serious consequences.

So what should we do? There are three alternatives I have heard of, and there may well be more. The first one is *laissez faire*: just continue to enjoy the twenty-first century while it lasts, and I suspect this is what will happen. Secondly, the high-tech road: take environmental problems seriously and replace fossil fuel energy as soon as possible with renewable energy, and I would suggest with nuclear energy; encourage the chemical and biochemical industries to supply our food needs by synthesis from inorganic raw materials; and then, finally, go vegetarian, because this would greatly increase the yield of available food from farmland. Entirely visionary. The third is the deep green way: eat nothing but organic food; use nothing but renewable energy and raw materials; and use alternative rather than scientific medicine. This would probably succeed in a massive reduction in the world population. All three approaches coexist in the first world, and the present state of environmental awareness worldwide reminds me very much of the UK in the 1930s. We suspected then that there would be another world war, but we were very confused about what to do about it. As in those times, I suspect little will be done unless and until there is a global mishap, for example a sudden rise of sea level sufficient to threaten major cities.

Dayan: I hadn't meant that to be quite a closing statement, but it is a set of very profound thoughts. Shall we stop with those ideas in our minds? Thank you very much everybody for contributing so very helpfully and freely.

Dr Daphne Christie: I would like to thank you all for participating in this afternoon's seminar. It has been very interesting to listen to your recollections and to hear your debates. May I add my particular thanks to Professor Dayan for the excellent chairing of this meeting and I hope you will join me in thanking him. Thank you very much.

---

[216] See Watson (2001).

References

Ackermann-Liebrich U, Rapp R. (1999) Epidemiological effects of oxides of nitrogen, especially NO_2. Ch. 25, in Holgate S T, Samet J M, Koren H S, Maynard R L. (eds) *Air Pollution and Health*. San Diego: Academic Press, 561–84.

Advisory Committee on Pesticides. (2002) *Annual Report 2002*. London: Department for Environment, Food and Rural Affairs.

Advisory Group on the Medical Aspects of Air Pollution Episodes. (1991) *Ozone: First report of the Advisory Group on the Medical Aspects of Air Pollution Episodes*. London: HMSO.

Altenburger R. (1993) Pesticides in EC drinking water – limit value may be raised. *Pesticides News* **22**: 10.

Ames B, Lee F, Durston W. (1973) An improved bacterial test system for the detection and classification of mutagens and carcinogens. *Proceedings of the National Academy of Sciences* **70**: 782–86.

Ames B, Haroun L, Andrews A W, Thibault L H, Lijinsky W. (1979) The reliability of the Ames assay for the prediction of chemical carcinogenicity. *Mutation Research* **62**: 393–99.

Amron D M, Moy R L. (1991) Stratospheric ozone depletion and its relationship to skin cancer. *Journal of Dermatologic Surgery and Oncology* **17**: 370–72.

Anderson H R. (1999) Health effects of air pollution episodes. Ch 21, in Holgate S T, Samet J M, Koren H S, Maynard R L. (eds) *Air Pollution and Health*. San Diego: Academic Press, 461–82.

Anonymous. (1983) Opren scandal. *Lancet* **i**: 219–20.

Ashby J, de Serres F J, Selby M D, Margolin B H, Ishidate M, Becking G C. (eds) (1988) *Evaluation of Short-term Tests for Carcinogens*, 2 vols. Cambridge: Cambridge University Press.

Barnes J M, Stoner H B. (1959) The toxicology of tin compounds. *Pharmacological Reviews* **11**: 211–31.

Bayer R. (ed.) (1988) Introduction. *The Health and Safety of Workers: Case studies in the politics of professional responsibility.* New York: Oxford University Press, 5–6.

Bazalgette J. (1864–5) The main drainage of London. *Minutes of Proceedings, Institution of Civil Engineers* 24: 285.

Beal S, Blundell H. (1978) Sudden infant death syndrome related to position in the cot. *Medical Journal of Australia* 2: 217–18.

Berridge V, Taylor S. (2002) *The Big Smoke: Fifty years after the 1952 London smog – A commemorative conference.* London: London School of Hygiene & Tropical Medicine.

Berry C. (2002) Nonsense and non-science. *Quarterly Journal of Medicine* 95: 131–2.

Booth W H, Kershaw J B C. (1904) *Smoke Prevention and Fuel Economy.* London: A Constable and Co. Ltd.

Boyer P. (2001) *Religion Explained: The human instincts that fashion gods, spirits and ancestors.* London: Heinemann.

Bray W. (ed.) (1890) *The Diary of John Evelyn, Esq., F.R.S.: from 1641 to 1705–6, with memoir.* London, New York: F Warne.

Brimblecombe P. (1987) *The Big Smoke: A history of air pollution in London since medieval times.* London: Routledge.

British Medical Association. (1990) *Pesticides, Chemicals and Health.* London: Edward Arnold.

Brooks P. (1980) Carson, Rachel Louise, in Sicherman B, Green C H. (eds) *Notable American Women. The Modern Period. A Biographical Dictionary.* Cambridge, USA and London: The Belknap Press of Harvard University Press.

Campbell E J M. (1965) Respiratory failure. *British Medical Journal* i: 1451.

Carson R. (1962) *Silent Spring.* Boston: Houghton Mifflin; London: Hamish Hamilton, 1963.

Chadwick E. (1842) *Report on the Sanitary Condition of the Labouring Population of Great Britain.* London: HMSO.

Committee on Air Pollution. (1958) *Report.* London: HMSO.

Committee on the Medical Effects of Air Pollutants. (1995) *Asthma and Outdoor Air Pollution.* London: HMSO.

Condit C. (2001) What is 'public opinion' about genetics? *Nature Reviews in Genetics* 2: 811–15.

Cox R A, Eggleton A E J, Derwent R G, Lovelock J E, Pack D H. (1975) Long-range transport of photochemical ozone in north-western Europe. *Nature* 255: 118–21.

Davies J E. (1982) Sleeping sickness and the factors affecting it in Botswana. *Journal of Tropical Medicine and Hygiene* 85: 63–71.

Dawkins R. (1986) *The Blind Watchmaker.* Harlow: Longman Scientific and Technical.

De Lemos M L. (2001) Effects of soy phytoestrogens genistein and daidzein on breast cancer growth. *Annals of Pharmacotherapy* 35: 1118–1121.

Dennett D. (1995) *Darwin's Dangerous Idea: Evolution and the meanings of life.* New York: Simon and Schuster.

Department of Health (DoH). (1998) *Report: Quantification of the effects of air pollution on health in the United Kingdom.* Committee on the Medical Effects of Air Pollutants (COMEAP). London: HMSO.

DoH. (2001) *Statement and Report on Long-term Effects of Particles on Mortality.* Committee on the Medical Effects of Air Pollutants. London: HMSO.

Department of Health and Social Security, Working Party on Lead in the Environment. (1980) *Lead and Health: The report of a DHSS Working Party on Lead in the Environment.* London: HMSO. Chairman, P J Lawther.

Department of the Environment (DoE). (1977) *Environmental Mercury and Man,* Pollution Paper no. 10. London: HMSO.

DoE. (1980) *Cadmium in the Environment and its Significance to Man,* Pollution Paper no. 17. London: HMSO.

DoE. (1994) *Expert Panel on Air Quality Standards: Benzene.* London: HMSO.

DoE, Central Unit on Environmental Pollution. (1974) *Non-Agricultural Uses of Pesticides in Great Britain: A report by the Central Unit on Environmental Pollution, Department of Environment,* Pollution Paper no. 3. London: HMSO.

Department of the Environment, Transport and the Regions. (1999) *The Government's Chemicals Strategy: Sustainable production and use of chemicals – a strategic approach.* London: Department of the Environment, Transport and the Regions.

DeWitt J. (1955) Effects of chlorinated hydrocarbon insecticides upon quail and pheasants. *Journal of Agriculture and Food Chemistry* 3: 672–6.

DeWitt J. (1956) Chronic toxicity to quail and pheasants of some chlorinated insecticides. *Journal of Agriculture and Food Chemistry* 4: 863–6.

Doll R. (1995) The first reports on smoking and lung cancer, in Lock S P, Reynolds L A, Tansey E M. (eds) *Ashes to Ashes: The history of smoking and health.* Amsterdam: Rodopi, 1998.

Dunlap T R. (1981) *DDT: Scientists, citizens and public policy.* Princeton: Princeton University Press.

Dupont B J Jr, Cohn I Jr. (1980) Gastric adenocarcinoma. *Current Problems in Cancer* 4: 1–46.

EEC. (1993) Directive on evaluation and control of risks of existing substances. Council Regulation (EEC) 793/93.

EEC. (1967) Directive relating to the classification, packaging and labelling of dangerous substances, as amended. Council Directive 67/538/EEC.

Ehrlich P R. (1971) *The Population Bomb.* London: Ballantine Books.

Eldridge N, Gould S J. (1972) Punctuated equilibria: An alternative to phyletic gradualism, in Schopf T M. (ed.) *Models in Paleobiology.* San Francisco: Freeman, Cooper and Co., 82–115.

Evelyn J. (1661) *Fumifugium: Or the incovenience of the aer and smoak of London dissipated.* Together with some remedies humbly proposed by J E[velyn] Esq. London: Printed by W Godbid for Gabriel Bedel & T Collins.

Farber S M, Wilson R H L. (eds) (1961) *The Air We Breathe: A study of man and his environment.* Springfield: Charles C Thomas.

Farman J C, Gardiner B G, Shanklin J D. (1985) Large losses of total ozone in Antarctica reveal seasonal ClO_x/NO_x interaction. *Nature* **315**: 207–10.

Farr W. (1856) Letter to the Registrar General. *17th Annual Report of the Registrar General. British Parliamentary Papers (BPP)* **xviii**.

Farr W. (1867–8) Report of the cholera epidemic of 1866 in England. *British Parliamentary Papers* **xxxvii**: 95.

Fleming P J, Gilbert R, Azaz Y, Berry P J, Rudd P T, Stewart A, Hall E. (1990) Interaction between bedding and sleeping position in the sudden infant death syndrome: A population-based case-control study. *British Medical Journal* **301**: 85–9.

Freese B. (2003) *Coal: A human history.* Oxford: Perseus Publishing.

Fuller J G. (ed.) (1977) *The Poison that Fell from the Sky.* New York: Random House.

Gough M. (1986) *Dioxin, Agent Orange: The facts.* New York: Plenum Press.

Grada C A. (1999) *Black '47 and Beyond: The great Irish famine in history, economy and memory.* Princeton: Princeton University Press.

Graebner W. (1988) Private power, private knowledge, and public health: Science, engineering and lead poisoning, 1900–70, in Bayer R. (ed.) *The Health and Safety of Workers: Case studies in the politics of professional responsibility.* New York: Oxford University Press, 15–71.

Griffiths J. (1962) *The Clean Air Act 1956 – Smoke Control Areas: A memorandum.* London: Association of Public Health Inspectors.

Gunter V J, Harris C K. (1998) Noisy winter: The DDT controversy in the years before *Silent Spring. Rural Sociology* **63**: 179–98.

Halliday S. (2001) Death and miasma in Victorian London: An obstinate belief. *British Medical Journal* **323**: 1469–71.

Hanley J. (2002) Edwin Chadwick and the poverty of statistics. *Medical History* **46**: 21–40.

Hansen J C. (1998) The human health programme under Arctic Monitoring and Assessment Program (AMAP). AMAP Human Health Group. *International Journal of Circumpolar Health* **57**: 280–91.

Harada M. (1995) Minamata disease: methylmercury poisoning in Japan caused by environmental pollution. *Critical Reviews in Toxicology* **25**: 1–24.

Hemminki K, Dipple A, Shuker D E G, Kadlubar F F, Segerback D, Bartsch H. (eds) (1994) *DNA Adducts: Identification and biological significance.* IARC Scientific Publications, no. 125. Lyon: IARC Press.

Holgate S T, Samet J M, Koren H S, Maynard R L. (eds) (1999) *Air Pollution and Health.* San Diego: Academic Press.

Hooper K. (1999) Breast Milk Monitoring Programs (BMMPs): World-wide early warning system for polyhalogenated POPs and for targeting studies in children's environmental health. *Environmental Health Perspectives* **107**: 429–30.

Hughes J D. (1994) *Pan's Travail: Environmental problems of the ancient Greeks and Romans.* Baltimore and London: Johns Hopkins University Press.

Hunter D. (1978) The Beaver Committee and the Clean Air Act 1956, in Hunter D. (ed.) *The Diseases of Occupations*, 6th edn. London: Hodder and Stoughton, 151–2.

Huxley J S. (1942) *Evolution: The modern synthesis.* London: George Allen and Unwin Ltd.

International Agency for Research on Cancer (IARC). (1980) Some metals and metallic compounds. *IARC Monograph*, vol. 23. Lyon: IARC Press.

IARC. (1993) Some naturally occurring substances: Food items and constituents, heterocyclic amines and mycotoxins. *IARC Monograph*, vol. 56. Lyon: IARC Press.

IARC. (1997) Polychlorinated dibenzo-para-dioxins and polychlorinated dibenzofurans. *IARC Summary and Evaluation* **69**: 33, 345.

International Maritime Organization. (1991) *London Dumping Convention: The first decade and beyond. Marine Environment Protection.* London: International Maritime Organization.

Jackson J. (1998) Cognition and the global Malaria Eradication Program. *Parassitologia* **40**: 193–216.

John Taylor Teachers Centre. (n.d.) *Public Health in Leeds, 1700–1850.* Leeds: John Taylor Teachers Centre.

Kinealy C. (1997) *A Death-dealing Famine: The great hunger in Ireland.* London: Pluto Press.

Kulling S E, Rosenberg B, Jacobs E, Metzler M. (1999) The phytoestrogens, coumoestrol and genistein, induce structural chromosomal aberrations in cultured human peripheral blood lymphocytes. *Archives of Toxicology* **73**: 50–4.

Lansdown R, Yule W. (eds) (1986) *Lead Toxicity: History and environmental impact.* Baltimore: Johns Hopkins University Press.

Lawther P J. (1961) Urban air pollution and its effects on man. Ch. 14, in Farber S M, Wilson R H L. (eds) *The Air We Breathe: A study of man and his environment.* Springfield: Charles C Thomas, 206–11.

Lawther P J, Commins B T, Waller R E. (1965) A study of polycyclicaromatic hydrocarbons in gasworks Retort houses. *British Journal of Industrial Medicine* **22**: 13–20.

Last J M. (1993) Global change: Ozone depletion, greenhouse warming and public health. *Annual Review of Public Health* **14**: 115–36.

Lock S P, Reynolds L A, Tansey E M. (eds) (1998) *Ashes to Ashes – The history of smoking and health.* Amsterdam: Rodopi B V. Reprinted 2003.

Lovelock J E. (1971) Air pollution and climatic change. *Atmospheric Environment* **5**: 403–11.

Lovelock J E. (1997) Midwife to the greens: The electron capture detector. *Microbiologia* **13**: 11–22.

Maddison D, Pearce D. (1999) Costing and health effects of poor air quality, in Holgate S T, Samet J M, Koren H S, Maynard R L. (eds) *Air Pollution and Health*. San Diego: Academic Press, 917–28.

Magari S R, Schwartz J, Williams P L, Hauser R, Smith T J, Christiani D C. (2002) The association between personal measurements of environmental exposure to particulates and heart rate variability. *Epidemiology* **13**: 305–10.

Mahboubi E, Kmet J, Cook P J, Day N E, Ghadirian P, Salmasizadeh S. (1973) Oesophageal cancer studies in the Caspian littoral of Iran: The Caspian cancer registry. *British Journal of Cancer* **28**: 197–214.

Marc B, Blanchet P, Boniol L. (2001) Domestic aerosol and flash fire: Warning from a fatal case. *Burns* **27**: 783–4.

Marston P, O'Neill S, Davies C. (2000) Four killed as train derails at 115mph. *Daily Telegraph*, 18 October 2000.

Mason B J. (ed.) (1990) *The Surface Waters Acidification Programme*. Cambridge: Cambridge University Press.

Maynard R L, Waller R. (1999) Carbon monoxide. Ch. 33, in Holgate S T, Samet J M, Koren H S, Maynard R L. (eds) (1999) *Air Pollution and Health*. San Diego: Academic Press, 749–96.

McGregor D B, Partensky C, Wilbourn J, Rice J M. (1998) An IARC evaluation of polychlorinated dibenzo-p-dioxins and polychlorinated dibenzofurans as risk factors in human carcinogenesis. *Environmental Health Perspectives* **106**: 755–60.

McGregor D B, Rice J M, Venitt S. (eds) (1999) *Use of short term and medium term tests for carcinogens. Data on genetic effects in carcinogenic hazard evaluation*. IARC Scientific Publications, no. 146. Lyon: IARC Press.

McLaughlin G A. (1973) History of pyrethrum, in Casida J E. (ed.) *Pyrethrum: The natural insecticide*. New York: Academic Press.

Melville H. (1962) *The Department of Scientific and Industrial Research*, New Whitehall Series no. 9. London: George Allen & Unwin Ltd.

Miller A B, Bartsch H, Boffetta P, Dragsted L, Vainio H. (eds) (2001) *Biomarkers in cancer chemoprevention.* IARC Scientific Publications, no. 154. Lyon: IARC Press.

Ministry of Health. (1954) *Mortality and Morbidity During the London fog of December 1952: Report by a committee of departmental officers and expert advisers appointed by the Minister of Health.* Series Report on Public Health and Medical Subjects, no. 95. London: HMSO.

Ministry of Housing and Local Government; Department of Health for Scotland. (1956) *Clean Air Act, 1956.* London: HMSO.

Moriarty F. (1988) *Ecotoxicology: The study of pollutants in ecosystems.* London: Academic Press.

Müller P H. (1948) Dichlorodiphenyltrichloroathan und neuere inzekticde. Nobel Lecture in *Les Prix Nobel en 1948.* Stockholm: Elsevier, 122–32.

Müller P H. (ed.) (1955) *The insecticide dichlorodiphenyltrichloroethane and its significance.* Vol. 1. Basel and Stuttgart: Birkhäuser Verlag.

Najera J A, Shidrawi G R, Gibson F D, Stafford J S. (1967) A large-scale field trial of malathion as an insecticide for antimalarial work in southern Uganda. *Bulletin of the World Health Organization* **36**: 913–35.

Neuberger A, Smith R L. (1982) Richard Williams Tecwyn. *Biographical Memoirs of Fellows of the Royal Society* **28**: 685–717.

North K, Golding J. (2000) A maternal vegetarian diet in pregnancy is associated with hypospadias. Avon Longitudinal Study of Pregnancy and Childhood. *British Journal of Urology International* **85**: 107–13.

Nriagu J O. (ed.) (1998) Health Effects, Part 2. *Vanadium in the Environment.* Chichester: Wiley-Interscience.

Packard R M. (1998) 'No other logical choice': Global malaria eradication and the politics of international health in the post-war era. *Parassitologia* **40**: 217–29.

Pesatori A C, Consonni D, Bachetti S, Zocchetti C, Bonzini M, Baccarelli A, Bertazzi P A. (2003) Short- and long-term morbidity and mortality in the population exposed to dioxin after the 'Seveso accident'. *Industrial Health* **41**: 127–38.

Pobel D, Riboli E, Cornee J, Hemon B, Guyader M. (1995) Nitrosamine, nitrate and nitrite in relation to gastric cancer: a case-control study in Marseille, France. *European Journal of Epimioliogy* **11**: 67–73.

Policy Commission on the Future of Farming and Food. (2002) *Farming and Food: A sustainable future.* London: UK Cabinet Office.

Quiroga V. (1990) Paul Hermann Müller 1948, in Fox D M, Meldrum M, Rezak I. (eds) *Nobel Laureates in Medicine or Physiology.* New York and London: Garland Publishing Inc., 416–19.

Ramazzini B. (ed.) (1700) *De Morbis Artificum Diatribe.* Mutinae: Typis A Capponi.

Ramazzini B. (ed.) (1705) *A Treatise of the Diseases of Tradesmen.* London: A Bell.

Reynolds L A, Tansey E M. (eds) (2001) Childhood Asthma and Beyond. *Wellcome Witnesses to Twentieth Century Medicine*, vol 11. London: The Wellcome Trust Centre for the History of Medicine at UCL.

Reynolds L A, Tansey E M. (eds) (2003) Foot and Mouth Disease: The 1967 outbreak and its aftermath. *Wellcome Witnesses to Twentieth Century Medicine*, vol 18. London: The Wellcome Trust Centre for the History of Medicine at UCL.

Ristaino J B, Groves C T, Parra G R. (2001) PCR amplification of the Irish potato famine pathogen from historic specimens. *Nature* **411**: 695–97.

Royal Commission on Sewage Disposal. (1902–15) *Report of the Commissioners appointed in 1898 to inquire and report what methods of treating and disposing of sewage (including any liquid from any factory or manufacturing process) may properly be adopted.* London: HMSO.

Russell B A. (1967, 1968, 1969) *The Autobiography of Bertrand Russell.* 3 vols, London: George Allen and Unwin; Boston and Toronto: Little Brown and Company (vols 1 and 2), New York: Simon and Schuster (vol. 3).

Russell E P. (1999) The strange career of DDT: Experts, federal capacity and environmentalism in World War II. *Technology and Culture* **40**: 770–96.

Russell E. (2001) *War and Nature: Fighting humans and insects with chemicals from World War I to* Silent Spring. Cambridge: Cambridge University Press.

Samet J M, Jaakkola J J K. (1999) The epidemiologic approach to investigating iutdoor pollution. Ch. 20, in Holgate S T, Samet J M, Koren H S, Maynard R L. (eds) *Air Pollution and Health*. San Diego: Academic Press, 431–60.

Schulze E-D, Lange O L, Oren R. (eds) (1989) *Forest Decline and Air Pollution: A study of spruce* (Picea abies) *on acid soils*. Berlin: Springer-Verlag.

Setchell K D R, Zimmer-Nechemias L, Cai J, Heubi J. (1997) Exposure of infants to phyto-oestrogens from soy-based infant formula. *Lancet* **350**: 23–27.

Sharpe R. (1988) *The Cruel Deception: The use of animals in medical research*. Wellingborough: Thorsons Publishing Group.

Smil V. (2001) *Enriching the Earth: Fritz Haber, Carl Bosch and the transformation of world food production*. Cambridge (USA) and London: MIT Press.

Tansey E M. (1993) The history of toxicology: The long and short of it. *Human and Experimental Toxicology* **12**: 459–61.

Tansey E M, Reynolds L A. (eds) (1997) The Committee on Safety of Drugs. *Wellcome Witnesses to Twentieth Century Medicine*, vol 1. London: The Wellcome Trust, 103–33.

Thomas K. (1983) *Man and the Natural World*. London: Allen Lane.

Thomas L. (1983) *The Youngest Science*. New York: Viking Press.

Thomas M R. (1997) *Pesticide Usage Survey Report 100: Review of usage of pesticides in agriculture and horticulture throughout Great Britain, 1984–94*. MAFF Reference Book PB 2943. London: MAFF Publications.

Toniolo P, Boffetta P, Shuker D E G, Rothman N, Hulka B, Pearce N. (eds) (1997) *Application of Biomarkers in Cancer Epidemiology*. IARC Scientific Publications, no. 142. Lyon: IARC Press.

Tren R, Bate R. (2001) *Malaria and the DDT Story*. London: Institute of Economic Affairs.

Turner B S. (1992) *Max Weber: From history to modernity*. London: Routledge.

Uhlig R. (2002) Farmers warn Beckett over EU manure mountains. *Daily Telegraph*, 12 March 2002.

United Nations Economic Commission for Europe. (1998) *Convention on Long-range Transboundary Air Pollution: Protocol on persistent organic pollutants*. New York and Geneva: United Nations.

Ward H. (2003) *A Man of Small Importance: My father Griffin Barry*. Debenham: Dormouse Books, 278.

Watson R T. (2001) *Climate Change 2001. Third Assessment Report of the Intergovernmental Panel on Climate Change*. Cambridge: Cambridge University Press.

Weber M. (1976) The Protestant ethic and the spirit of capitalism. *Die Protestantisch Arbeitsethik und der Geist von Kapitalismus* (1902) translated by T Parsons. 2nd edn. London: Allen & Unwin.

Whorton J. (1974) *Before* Silent Spring: *Pesticides and public health in pre-DDT America*. Princeton: Princeton University Press.

Wilkins E T. (1954) Air pollution and the London fog of December, 1952. *Journal of the Royal Sanitary Institute* 74: 1–21.

Williams R T. (1959) *Detoxication Mechanisms: The metabolism and detoxication of drugs, toxic substances and other organic compounds*. 2nd edn. London: Chapman and Hall.

Wilson E O. (2002) *The Future of Life*. New York: Alfred A Knopf.

Wohl A S. (1983) *Endangered Lives: Public health in Victorian and Edwardian England*. London and Cambridge: J M Dent and Harvard University Press.

Wolstenholme G, Luniewska V. (1984) Hunter, Donald. *Munk's Roll* 7: 288–90.

World Health Organization (WHO). (1972) *Air Quality Criteria and Guides for Urban Air Pollutants,* Report of a WHO Expert Committee. World Health Organization Technical Report Series no. 506. Geneva: WHO.

Zaporowska H, Wasilewski W. (1992) Haematological effects of vanadium on living organisms. *Comparative Biochemistry and Physiology* C **102**: 223–31.

Zhu Z-L, Wen Q-X, Freney J R. (eds) (1997) *Nitrogen in Soils of China.* Dordrecht: Kluwer Academic Publishers.

Biographical notes

Professor Bruce Ames

has been Professor of Biochemistry and Molecular Biology at the University of California, Berkeley, USA, and Director of the National Institute of Environmental Health Sciences Centre at the University of California. He was a member of the Board of Directors of the US National Cancer Institute, and its Advisory Board, from 1976 to 1982.

Sir Colin Berry

Kt HonFRCP FRCPath (b. 1937) qualified in medicine at the University of London in 1961, winning the Governors' Gold Medal. He became Lecturer at the Institute of Child Health, Great Ormond Street, London, and a British Heart Foundation Research Fellow. He was appointed Reader in Pathology at Guy's Hospital, London, in 1970 and Professor and Head of the Department of Morbid Anatomy at the Royal London Hospital in 1976. In 1994 he was elected Dean of the London Hospital Medical College, and from 1994 to 1996 was Warden of St Bartholomew's and the London Hospital Medical and Dental Hospital. He was a member of the Committee on the Safety of Medicines (1990–92) and Chairman of the Advisory Committee on Pesticides (1988–99).

Sir Christopher Booth

Kt FRCP (b.1924) trained as a gastroenterologist and was the first Convenor of the Wellcome Trust's History of Twentieth Century Medicine Group, from 1990 to 1996, and Harveian Librarian at the Royal College of Physicians from 1989 to 1997. He was Professor of Medicine, Royal Postgraduate Medical School, Hammersmith Hospital, London, from 1966 to 1977 and Director of the Medical Research Council's Clinical Research Centre, Northwick Park Hospital, Harrow, from 1978 to 1988.

Professor Moran Campbell

became Assistant Professor at the Medical Unit of the Middlesex Hospital in 1955. He went on to hold the first Chair of Medicine at McMaster University, Kingston, Canada, and is now Emeritus Professor of Medicine, Division of Respirology at the Department of Medicine there.

Rachel Carson

FRSL (1907–64) studied biology at Johns Hopkins University, taught at the University of Maryland (1931–6) and worked as a marine biologist for the US Fish and Wildlife Service (1936–49). During the Second World War she wrote conservation bulletins for the government. Her influential book, *Silent Spring* (1962), drew attention to the dangers inherent in the use of DDT and other toxic chemicals. The resulting controls in the USA on the use of pesticides owed much to her work, which also contributed to the increasing ecological and conservationist attitudes that emerged in the 1970s. See Brooks (1980).

Professor Richard Carter

CBE FRCP FRCPath (b. 1934) qualified in medicine at Oxford in 1960 and was a clinical and experimental histopathologist at the Royal Marsden Hospital, London, and Institute of Cancer Research between 1974 and 2001 as Honorary Consultant and Reader. He was Honorary Professor at the University of Surrey (1994–2002), has served on various advisory committees for government departments, and was Chairman of the Carcinogenicity Committee at the Department of Health (1985–95).

Dr Peter Corcoran

(b. 1939) trained as a physicist and later worked for the Department of Environment from 1971 until his retirement in 1999. From 1980 to 1999 he was head of a unit in the Chemicals and Biotechnology Division of the Department of Environment responsible for policy on new and existing chemicals and pesticides. He was the Head of the UK Delegation to the OECD Chemicals Group (1987–99) and represented the UK in the negotiation of UN conventions on international trade in chemicals and persistent organic pollutants.

Professor Anthony Dayan

FRCP FRCPath FIBiol (b. 1935) was Professor of Toxicology at St Bartholomew's Hospital Medical College, London, from 1984 to 1998. He had also worked in the NHS and in the pharmaceutical industry. His particular interest is the relationship between the uncertainties of science and the certainties of government regulation.

Professor Peter Farmer

FRCS CChem (b. 1947) spent much of his research career in the MRC Toxicology Unit, first in Carshalton and later in Leicester. Since 2002 he has been Joint Director of the MRC Cancer Biomarkers and Prevention ESS (external scientific staff) Group at the University of Leicester. He is an Honorary Professor in Biochemistry and Cancer Studies at the University of Leicester and has been Chairman of the Government Advisory Committee on

Mutagenicity of Chemicals in Food, Consumer Products and the Environment, since 2001.

Dr Robert Flanagan

CChem FRSC FRCPath (b. 1948) has worked in clinical and forensic analytical toxicology since 1970. He has acted as adviser to the United Nations International Drug Programme, the International Programme on Chemical Safety, and the UK National Crime and Operations Faculty on aspects of analytical toxicology.

Dr Donald Hunter

CBE FRCP (1898–1978) was Consulting Physician to the London Hospital from 1927 to 1963 and Director of the MRC Department for Research in Industrial Medicine at the London Hospital from 1943 to 1963. He was the Founding Editor of the *British Journal of Industrial Medicine* from 1944. See Wolstenholme and Luniewska (1984).

Dr Peter Hunter

(b. 1938) qualified from Middlesex Hospital, London, in 1963 and was Consultant Physician at the Royal Shrewsbury Hospital, specializing in endocrinology, from 1974 to 1993. From 1994 to 1997 he read pharmacology at King's College London, as preparation for research on the history of drug discovery in the modern era.

Mr Stanley Johnson

(b. 1940) was former Head of the European Commission's Prevention of Pollution and Nuisances Division, and former MEP and Vice-Chairman of the European Parliament's Committee on the Environment, Public Health and Consumer Protection.

Professor Patrick (Pat) Lawther

CBE FRCP (b. 1921) was Professor of Environmental and Preventative Medicine, University of London, at St Bartholomew's Hospital Medical College from 1968 to 1981 and at London Hospital Medical College from 1976 to 1981. He was a member of the Medical Research Council Scientific Staff from 1955 to 1981 and directed the MRC Air Pollution Unit (later the Environmental Hazards Unit) from 1955 to 1977.

Professor James Lovelock

CH CBE FRS (b. 1919) was a member of staff of the National Institute for Medical Research, London, from 1941 to 1964. From 1964 he has been an independent scientist working from his home laboratory. He was President of the Marine Biological Association from 1986 to 1991 and since 1990 he has been a visiting fellow of Green College, Oxford.

Professor Robert Maynard
CBE FRCP FRCPath FFOM
(b. 1951) has been Senior Medical Officer and Head of the Air Pollution Team at the UK Department of Health since 1990. He was Medical Secretary to the Committee on the Medical Effects of Air Pollutants and to the Expert Panel on Air Quality Standards, Editor of the World Health Organization's *Air Quality Guidelines* for Europe and has been Honorary Professor in the Institute of Public Health at Birmingham University, since 2000.

Professor Ingar Palmlund
(b. 1938) was Director of the Swedish Council of Environmental Information from 1973 to 1977. After a career as a senior civil servant in Sweden she returned to academia as Associate Professor at the Department of Technology and Social Change, at Linköping University, Sweden and lectures on international environmental policy at Tufts University, Medford, USA.

Dr Leslie Reed
(b. 1925) worked in the Central Unit on Environmental Pollution, Department of the Environment from 1970 to 1979. He became Head of the Air and Noise Division from 1979 to 1981, and Chief Industrial Air Pollution Inspector, Health and Safety Executive, from 1981 to 1985.

Dr Dennis Simms
(b. 1926) joined the Central Unit for Environmental Protection (CUEP) in 1972 to run the London Dumping Conference, and subsequently was Secretary to the Interim Paris Committee on Land Pollution (1972–77). He was member of the UK Delegation to the UN Third Law of the Sea Conference and leader of the Third Committee on Preservation of Marine Environment. His responsibility covered a wide range of environmental problems and developed ideas on risk assessment. He was also Chairman of the Advisory Committee to European Commission on environmental protection research and development from 1985 to 1987.

Professor Robert Smith
was Head of the Division of Biomedical Sciences, Imperial College of Science, Technology and Medicine, London (1976–92), now Emeritus Professor, and is a past member of the Committee on Safety of Medicines.

Professor Richard Tecwyn Williams
FRS (1909–79) was Professor of Biochemistry at St Mary's Hospital Medical School, London, from 1949 to 1976, and Dean from 1970 to 1976. Following Sir Archibald Garrod's work on the role of enzymes in drug metabolism,

Williams developed detoxication chemistry as a science in its own right, and established the two-phase drug metabolism in animals. In 1931 he published the structure of gluconuronic acid, and spent the rest of his career examining the fate of foreign compounds in the body. See Neuberger and Smith (1982).

Professor H Frank Woods
CBE FRCP FRCPE FFPM
(b. 1937) is the Sir George Franklin Professor of Medicine and Director of the Division of Clinical Sciences (South), and served as Dean of the Faculty of Medicine (1988–98), University of Sheffield. He was awarded a CBE for his services to the Committee on Toxicity of Chemicals in Food, Consumer Products and the Environment. He was formerly Chairman of the General Medical Council's Health Committee.

Glossary

Note the use of bold for items in glossary.

1,1-bis(4-chlorophenyl)-2,2,2-trichloroethane (DDT)

A persistent fat-soluble insecticide that has been used against a wide variety of insects. Its use was banned in the USA in 1972, and in the UK in 1986.

Acrolein

A pungent colourless unsaturated liquid aldehyde used in the manufacture of resins and pharmaceuticals.

Aflatoxin

Any of a group of chemically-related fungal metabolites produced by some strains of *Aspergillus flavus* and *A. parasiticus*, commonly found in nuts and grains. It has been implicated in the causation of liver-cell carcinomas.

Aldrin

A polycyclic chlorinated hydrocarbon used as an insecticide, but toxic to mammals. The UK Environmental Protection Agency banned its use in 1987.

Bordeaux mixture

A common agricultural and horticultural fungicide consisting of a solution of equal quantities of copper sulphate and calcium hydroxide. It is used in the control of *Phytophthora infestans* (late potato blight).

Carcinogen

A cancer-causing substance or action.

Chlorofluorocarbon (CFC)

Any of various gaseous compounds of carbon, hydrogen, chlorine, bromine and fluorine used as refrigerants, aerosol propellants, solvents and in foam, which are implicated in the greenhouse effect.

Coumarin

A white vanilla-scented crystalline ester, used in perfumes and flavourings and as an anticoagulant.

Cyanobacteria

A group of photosynthetic bacteria formerly known as cyanophytes or blue-green algae.

DDT

See **1,1-bis(4-chlorophenyl)-2,2,2-trichloroethane**.

Dieldrin

A long-lasting chlorinated hydrocarbon, used to control mosquitoes, ticks, sand flies and other agricultural and forest pests. The Environmental Protection Agency banned its use in 1987.

Dioxin
A toxic chlorinated hydrocarbon often present as a contaminant in the preparation of 2,4,5-T, a widely used herbicide.

Emetine
Methylcephaeline, an alkaloid that has been used to treat schistosomiasis.

Genistein
A naturally occurring substance in soya beans and other plants with oestrogen-like actions.

Greenhouse effect
A process by which levels of some gases in the planet's atmosphere results in a higher temperature than the planet would have otherwise.

Hypospadias
A developmental defect of the urethra in which the urethral folds fail to unite to complete the ventral wall of the urethra.

Ipecacuanha
Ipecac, a substance used as an emetic drug.

Malathion
The first commercial **organophosphate** pesticide to come on to the market in 1950.

Oestriol
A metabolic product of oestradiol and oestrone found in mammalian urine, especially during pregnancy.

Organophosphates
Neurotoxins that can attack the nervous system used as pesticides for home and agricultural use. See **malathion**.

Paraquat
An extremely poisonous soluble solid used in solution as a weedkiller.

Pesticide
An agent used to control pests and diseases, including insecticides, herbicides and fungicides.

Pyrethrin
Any of the esters of chrysanthemum dicarboxylic acid found in the dried flower heads of pyrethrum and which account for the insecticidal properties of pyrethrum. Widely adopted as an environmental friendly insecticide from the 1970s, although less effective than the **organophosphates**.

Teratogen
An agent or factor capable of causing developmental abnormality in an embryo or fetus, including radiation or viral infection, or a chemical or drug.

Tetraethyl lead

A toxic oily, colourless liquid, added to gasoline as an antiknocking agent. It is readily absorbed from car exhaust fumes through the skin and respiratory tract of mammals.

Toxicokinetics

The study of the rate of change of the concentration of harmful substances and any metabolites in an organism.

Trialkyltins

Simple chemicals, for example, tributyltin (TBT), containing tin bound to various alkyl groups containing carbon and hydrogen, which produce powerful fungicides, biocides and bactericides. Formerly used as antifouling agents (see page 31).

Venturi mask

A mask for oxygen inhalation that enables three different concentrations of inhaled oxygen, 24, 28 or 35 per cent, at different flow rates. Oxygen flows down a narrow tube and leaves the tube at reduced pressure. Air around the oxygen stream is sucked into it thereby reducing the oxygen concentration. See Campbell (1965).

Xenotransplantation

An operation in which an organ or tissue is transferred from one animal to another of a different species.

Index: Subject

1,1-bis(4-chlorophenyl)-2,2,2-
  trichloroethane *see* DDT
acid rain, 42–5
acrolein, 54, 95
Advisory Committee on Pesticides
  (ACP), 8
aerosol propellants, 28
aflatoxin (B1), 68, 95
Agent Orange, 33
agriculture
  benefits of modern, 6–7
  future policy, 62, 72
  use of pesticides, 3–4, 11, 61–2
  water pollution, 21, 60–1
air pollution, 10, 38, 42–8, 52–7
  analytical methods, 5
  cost–benefit analysis, 48, 52, 54–6
  early history, 52–3
  effects of very low concentrations,
    63–4, 66–7
  European cities, 56, 59, 60
  health impact, 46–8, 53, 54, 63, 66–7
  motor traffic-generated, 53, 54, 59
  particulate, 48, 53
  transboundary problems, 42–5
Air Pollution Research Unit, MRC,
  London, 46
The Air We Breathe (Farber and Wilson;
  1961), 47
Alar, 36
aldehydes, 54
aldrin, 27, 39, 95
Alkali Act, 54, 63
Alkali Inspectorate, 54, 63
allergy, 67
aluminium sulphate, 51
Amazonian forest, 7
Ames test, 26–7, 30

Amoco Cadiz incident (1978), France, 34
analytical methods, 5–6, 69
  vs biological effects, 17, 18
  wet chemical, 5
animals
  attitudes to use in research, 26
  carcinogenicity testing, 70, 71
  toxicity testing, 10
  see also cattle
apples, 36
  see also Alar
Arctic, 39
arsenic salts, 68
arsine, Market Drayton accident
  (1975), 36
asbestos, 38, 41
Aspergillus flavus, 68
asthma, 53
Athens, 56, 59, 60
atrazine, 35
Auschwitz, 4
Australia, 6, 16

Baltic Convention, 62
Bari harbour mustard gas disaster
  (1943), 36
Basel Convention (1989), 41
Beaver Committee, 46
benoxaprofen (Opren), 11
benzene, 19, 70, 71
Bhopal accident (1984), India, 34
Bight of Benin, 15
'biological toxicology,' 20
biomarkers, 17, 25, 64, 71
birds, 5, 11, 13
blue-baby syndrome, 21
Bordeaux mixture, 3–4, 95
Botswana, 12

bovine spongiform encephalopathy (BSE), 20, 62
Bradshaw's Guide, 60
British Antarctic Survey (BAS), 28
British Medical Association (BMA), 67
Brittany, *Amoco Cadiz* incident (1978), 34
bronchitis, chronic, 63
BSE *see* bovine spongiform encephalopathy
butane, 28

cadmium, 37
California Proposition 65, 72
Camelford water-poisoning incident (1988), Cornwall, 51
Canada, 39, 63
cancer
    President Nixon's war against, 24
    risks, concerns about, 13–14, 22–4
    see also carcinogens
car emissions, 53, 54, 55–6
carbon dioxide (CO_2)
    chronic retention, 63
    greenhouse effect, 15
carbon monoxide, 54
carcinogenesis, 25–7, 69
carcinogens, 67–72, 95
    air-borne, 48
    genotoxic, 25, 26–7, 58, 69, 71
    increasing concerns over, 13–14, 26
    nongenotoxic, 25, 58, 69–70
    public perceptions, 22–4
    regulatory control, 71–2
    risk assessment, 70–2
    testing procedures, 69–70, 71
    water-borne, 51
catalytic converters, 54
cattle
    deaths in great smog (1952), 38, 45–6
    slurry farming, 60
Central Middlesex Hospital, London, 63

Central Unit (later Directorate) for Environmental Protection (CUEP), 37, 38
Centre Kleber, Paris, 64
Ceylon (now Sri Lanka), 9
CFCs *see* chlorofluorocarbons
Chadwickian (sanitary) movement, 49–50, 63
chemical industry, 27–9, 37
chemical plants
    accidents, 32–4
    European regulation, 32, 33
chemicals
    international agreements, 39–42
    low concentrations, 5–6, 18–20
    regulatory control, 10, 29–30, 42
    see also analytical methods, pesticides, health effects
chemistry departments, university, 32
children
    toxic effects of lead, 36
    see also infants
chimneys, raised height, 42
China, 7, 29
Chisso Corporation, 36
chlorofluorocarbons (CFCs), 5, 21, 57, 95
    removal from unwanted fridges, 34
    response of industry, 27–8
classical times, 3
Clean Air Act, 1956, 42, 46, 53, 63
climate change, global (global warming), 14–15, 37, 54, 57, 72–3
climatologists, 14–15
clinical ecology, 66, 67
coal burning, 38, 45, 46, 52, 53
Coal Smoke Abatement Society, 52
coal-tar dyes, 3
coffins, shortage of, 52
Committee on the Medical Effects of Air Pollutants, 67

Committee on Toxicity (COT), 24, 64
Convention on Long-range
    Transboundary Air Pollution, 44
Convention on the Prevention of
    Marine Pollution by Dumping of
    Wastes and Other Matters (London
    Dumping Convention; 1972), 61, 62
Cost–benefit analysis, 59–60
    air pollution, 48, 52, 54–6
    water quality standards, 21, 56
    see also risk–benefit analysis
cost–effectiveness analysis, 55
coumarin, 72, 95
Council of Europe, 65
crops
    pest-related losses, 7
    selective breeding, 7
Curry Report (2001), 62
cyanobacteria, 7, 95

Daily Telegraph, 21
DDT, 4, 8–9, 29, 39, 95
    analytical methods, 5–6
    risk–benefit analysis, 11–12
decision-making process
    open vs closed discussion, 24–5, 36
    scientific input, 8, 14
    water quality standards, 20–1
Delaney Clause (1958), 23–4, 25, 26
Denmark, 9
Department of Environment (DoE)
    Central Unit (later Directorate) for
        Environmental Protection, 37, 38
    Clean Air Act and, 53
    Toxic Substances Division, 31
Department of Health (DoH), 66
Department of Health and Human
    Services (DHHS), USA, 26
Department of Transport, 55
Detoxication Mechanisms (Williams;
    1959), 19

developing world, 29, 39, 40–1
diarrhoea, water-borne, 60–1
dieldrin, 5–6, 27, 39, 95
diesel vehicle emissions, 54, 59
dimethylsulphide, 43
dioxins, 39, 40, 96
    Seveso accident (1976), 32–4
    used in Vietnam, 33
disasters, environmental, 32–5, 36–7
The Diseases of Workmen (Ramazzini;
    1705), 68
dose thresholds, 19, 25, 47
dose–response relationships (curves),
    9–10, 19
    extrapolation to low doses, 19, 67,
        70–1
    at low doses, 58, 59, 63–4, 66–7
Doulton's pottery, and hydrochloric
    acid, 46
drugs, genetic make-up and, 11

ECE *see* Economic Commission for
    Europe
Economic Commission for Europe
    (ECE; UNECE), 39, 44
economics
    monitoring water quality, 50–1
    Stockholm Convention, 40
    toxicological testing, 29
    see also cost–benefit analysis
Edward I, King, 53
EEC *see* European Union
electricity-generating plants, 44–5
electron capture detector (ECD), 5
emetine, 4, 96
emissions
    motor vehicles, 53, 54, 55–6, 59
    regulatory control of industrial, 33,
        42, 44, 54
    into rivers and seas, 65–6
endocrine disturbances, 14

endosulfan, 12
endrin, 39
energy resources, 72, 73
entzauberung, 9
environment
    attitudes to, 8–9, 12–14, 15
    natural, 68–9
    vs neo-Darwinism, 18
environmental disasters, 32–5, 36–7
    see also Seveso accident, Bhopal
        accident, Market Drayton accident
Environmental Protection Agency
    (EPA), 5, 27, 30, 60
EPA see Environmental Protection
    Agency
epidemiological studies, 59, 63–4, 66
EU see European Union
European Union (EU; formerly
    European Economic Community;
    EEC)
    banning of trialkyltins, 31
    ENV 131 draft directive, 65
    environmental and product
        standards, 10
    environmental programme, 9–10, 15
    fridge mountain, 34, 57
    Registration, Evaluation and
        Authorization of Chemicals
        (REACH) policy, 30
    regulation of air pollution, 44–5
    regulation of existing chemicals, 10,
        29, 30, 42
    regulation of new chemicals (1967
        sixth amendment), 10, 29–30, 42
    regulation of toxic waste, 34
    Seveso directive, 32, 33–4
    water framework directive, 66
    water quality standards, 20–1, 35,
        51, 57–8, 65–6

Falklands Islands Dependencies Survey, 28
FAO (Food and Agriculture
    Organization), 15
farming see agriculture
fish, 36, 51, 58, 60
fogs, 52, 63
food
    chemical contamination, 58
    production, 72, 73
    spoilage/toxins, 7
Food, Drug and Cosmetic Bill, Delaney
    amendment (1958), 23–4, 25, 26
Food and Agriculture Organization
    (FAO), 15
foot and mouth disease, 62
forest die-back, in Germany, 44–5
formaldehyde, 54
France, 31, 34, 64–5
fridge mountain, 34, 57
Friends of the Earth, 57
FSID News, Foundation for the Study
    of Infant Deaths, 16
Fuel Research Station, Greenwich, 38, 53
Fumifugium, or, the inconvenience of the
    aer and smoake of London dissipated
    (Evelyn; 1661), 52
fungicides, 3–4

genistein, 22, 96
genotoxic carcinogens, 25, 26–7, 58,
    69, 71
Germany
    ban on methyl eugenol, 71
    forest die-off, 44–5
    see also Waldsterben
global warming see climate change,
    global
gold mining, 3
Green Issues, 14
greenhouse effect, 96
greenhouse gases, 12, 15, 21

Kyoto treaty (1997), 57
Greenpeace, 57

habitat loss, 72, 73
Hatfield train crash (October 2000), 17
hazard, 23, 71–2
HCFCs *see* hydrochlorofluorocarbons
health effects
    agriculture without pesticides, 7
    air pollution, 46–8, 53, 54, 63, 66–7
    assessment methods, 10
    concerns about, 8–10, 15
    cost–benefit analysis and, 55
    dose–response relationships *see*
      dose–response relationships
    risk assessment, 11–12, 18, 48, 70–2
    Seveso accident, 32
    vs environmental effects, 21
    water pollution, 60–1, 63
heart-rate variability, 66–7
herbicides, 4–5, 35, 62
homeopathic medicines, 6
hormones, in environment, 14
hydrochlorofluorocarbons (HCFCs), 57
hypospadias, 22, 96

I G Farben, and organophosphate
    pesticides, 4
IARC (International Agency for
    Research on Cancer), 15, 25
ICI, 28
ICMESA (Industrie Chimiche
    Mendionali Società Azionaria), 34
IMO (International Maritime
    Organization) Convention, 61
incineration, 39, 40, 59
India, 29, 34, 41
indicator species, 16
Industrial Revolution, 3
Industrie Chimiche Mendionali Società
    Azionaria (ICMESA), 34

industry
    chemical, 27–9, 37
    regulation of emissions, 33, 42, 44, 54
infants
    blue-baby syndrome, 21
    male, dangers of soya protein, 22
    sleeping position, 16
Inspector of Factories, 38
Intergovernmental Panel on Climate
    Change (IPCC), 72–3
International Agency for Research on
    Cancer (IARC), 15, 25
international conventions/agreements,
    15, 37–8, 39–42
    marine pollution, 61, 62–3, 64–5
International Maritime Organization
    (IMO) Convention, 61
International Programme on Chemical
    Safety (IPCS), 15
International Register of Potentially
    Toxic Chemicals (IRPTC), 42
IPCC (Intergovernmental Panel on
    Climate Change), 72–3
IPCS (International Programme on
    Chemical Safety), 15
ipecacuanha, 96
Iran, 68
Ireland, 9, 60
    potato famine (1845), 3
IRPTC (International Register of
    Potentially Toxic Chemicals), 42
Italy, Po Valley pollution, 35, 37

Japan, 36–7
Johannesburg, South Africa, 41
Joint Meeting on Pesticide Residues
    (JMPR), 15

Kyoto treaty (1997), 57

lakes, Scandinavian, 14, 42–5

Lancet, 19
land use changes, 6–7
Law of the Sea Convention (1982), 61, 62
lead
    in petrol, 38, 39
    toxicity, 3, 36
    see also children
lead arsenate, 3
Leeds, 49
leukaemias, 70
lice, 4
lions, 3
London
    air pollution, 45–6, 48, 52–3, 54,
        56, 59, 60, 63
    great smog (1952), 38, 45, 48, 52
    sewers, 49, 63
    water pollution, 49—50, 63
London Dumping Convention (1972),
    61, 62
London Evening Standard, 56
lung cancer, 48
lung disease, chronic, 63

Maastricht Treaty (1992), 9
malaria control, 4, 9, 39
malathion, 4, 96
    see also organophosphates
malformations, congenital, 33
Man and the Natural World (Thomas;
    1983), 13
manure, 21
marine pollution
    international conventions, 61, 62–3,
        64–5
    major incidents, 34, 36–7
    sewage, 58, 62
Market Drayton arsine accident (1975),
    36
McMaster University, Ontario, Canada,
    63
media, mass, 27

environmental carcinogens, 22–3
    presentation of scientific evidence,
        23, 35–6, 37
Medical History, 64
Medical Research Council (MRC), 8
    Air Pollution Research Unit, 46
    Systems Board, 16
Mediterranean Convention on the
    Prevention of Marine Pollution, 62–3
melanoma, malignant, 22
mercury poisoning, 36–7
methaemoglobin, 21
methodology, science, 15–16, 17, 18, 30
methyl chloroform, 27–8
methyl eugenol, 71
methyl isocyanate, 34
methyl mercury poisoning, 36
Minamata disease, 36–7
mining hazards, 3
molecular epidemiology, 69
Montreal protocol, 28
motor vehicle emissions, 53, 54, 55–6, 59
MRC *see* Medical Research Council
multiple chemical sensitivity, 66, 67
mustard gas, Bari harbour disaster
    (1943), 36
mutagenicity tests, 25, 30

National Institute for Medical
    Research, Mill Hill, London, 5
National Institute of Environmental
    Health Sciences (NIEHS), 26
National Society for Clean Air (now
    National Society for Clean Air and
    Environmental Protection), 57
National Toxicology Program (NTP),
    26, 71
Native Peoples Bureau, 39
natural environments, 68–9
Nature, 28
Nature Reviews in Genetics, 15–16
neo-Darwinism, 18

nicotine, 3
nitrates in water, 20–1, 23, 51, 57–8
nitrogen
    artificial, 7
    fixation, 6
nitrogen dioxide, 54
Nobel Prize, 4
nongenotoxic carcinogens, 25, 58, 69–70
Norway, dying lakes, 14, 42–5
Norwegian Pollution Control Agency, 14
NTP (National Toxicology Program),
    26, 71
nuclear energy, 73

occupational exposure, 68, 70, 71
OECD (Organization for Economic
    Cooperation and Development), 30, 42
oesophageal cancer, 68
oestriol, 96
    plasma, 22
oil, 38
    companies, 27, 37
    pollution, 34, 61
Opren, 11
Organization for Economic
    Cooperation and Development
    (OECD), 30, 42
organochlorine pesticides, 12, 19, 29
organophosphates, 4–5, 96
    see also malathion
Orissa, India, 41
Oslo Convention, 61, 62, 65
OSPAR Convention, 61
oxygen, 71
oysters, 31, 32
ozone
    atmospheric pollution, 59, 60
    layer (stratospheric) depletion, 12,
    21, 22, 27–8

paraquat, 35, 96

Paris Convention, 61, 62, 64–5
PCBs (polychlorinated biphenyls), 39
Persian Insect Powder, 4
persistent organic pollutants (POPs),
    29, 39–40, 41
pesticides, 3–42, 39, 96
    analytical methods see analytical
        methods
    awareness of environmental impact,
        12–13
    benefits, 6–7
    in drinking water, 51, 56, 61–2
    introduction, 3–5
    low concentrations, 5–6, 18–20
    multiple sources of exposure, 56, 64
    nonagricultural use, 61–2
    Po Valley contamination, 35
    regulatory control, 7–8
    response of industry, 27
    risk assessment, 11–12, 18
petrol, lead in, 38, 39
pheasant eggs, 11
phyto-oestrogens, 22
PIC (prior informed consent), 41
Po Valley, Italy, 35, 37
policy-making
    open vs closed discussion, 24–5
    precautionary principle see
        precautionary principle
    scientific input, 8, 14–15
    water quality standards, 20–1
'Pollution Papers,' 37
polychlorinated biphenyls (PCBs), 39
POPs (persistent organic pollutants),
    29, 39–40, 41
The Population Bomb (Ehrlich; 1971), 7
potato blight, 3
potteries, London, 46
precautionary principle, 16–17, 20, 24,
    39, 45, 72
prior informed consent (PIC), 41

public opinion
    acceptable risks, 11
    cancer risks, 22–4
    dioxins, 33
    influences on, 15–17, 18, 22–3,
        35–6, 37
    open decision-making and, 24–5, 36
punctuated equilibrium model of
    evolution, 18
pyrethrin, 4, 96
pyrethroid insecticides, 12
pyrethrum, 4

quail eggs, 11

Railway Workers' Union, 59
railways, 17, 59–60, 61
Registration, Evaluation and
    Authorization of Chemicals
    (REACH) policy, European Union, 30
reproductive hazards, 13–14, 25, 71
respiratory failure, 63
Rhine River, Germany, 65
risk
    acceptable, 11
    assessment, 11–12, 18, 48, 70–2
    vs hazard, 23, 71–2
    see also precautionary principle; zero
        tolerance
risk–benefit analysis, 11–12, 20
    see also cost–benefit analysis
rivers, 49–50, 60, 61
    see also Rhine, Thames
Roman Empire, 3
Russia, 6

sanitary movement, 49–50, 63
science
    in decision-making process, 8, 14–15
    improvements in understanding, 13
    methodology, 15–16, 17, 18, 30

presentation of results, 23, 35–6, 37
    public opinion and, 17, 24
scientists, 23
Sea Beirut, 41
sea pollution see marine pollution
Second World War, pesticide use
    during, 4, 8–9
selenium, 27
Seveso accident (1976), 32–4, 35, 38
Seveso directive, 32, 33–4
sewage, 49–50
    agricultural production, 60–1
    disposal in sea, 58, 62
sewers, London, 49, 63
Shell Centre, London, 27
ships
    antifouling agents, 31
    break-up for scrap, 41
    see also Sea Beirut
SIDS see sudden infant death syndrome
Silent Spring (Rachel Carson; 1962),
    12–14, 19–20, 72
    academic impact, 32
    apocalyptic view, 5, 6–7
    chronological context, 25, 26
    emphasis on birds, 11, 13
    environmental carcinogens and,
        13–14, 68, 69
    industry attitude, 27
    vs humanocentric attitudes, 8–9
silver mines, 3
slash and burn agriculture, 7
sleeping position, infants, 16
sleeping sickness, 12
slurry farming, 60
Smithfield Market, London, 45
smog
    great London, of 1952, 38, 45, 48, 52
    health impact, 63
    origin of term, 52
smokeless zones, 46

smoking, cigarette, 48
soya protein, 22
species, extrapolation across, 70
sperm counts, 22
St Bartholomew's Hospital, London, 46
Staines, Middlesex, 50
Stockholm Conference (1972) *see*
    United Nations Conference on the
    Human Environment, Stockholm
Stockholm Conference on the Human
    Environment (1972), 42, 61
Stockholm Convention (2001), 39–41
Stockholm Declaration (1972), 14
stomach carcinoma, 51
sudden infant death syndrome (SIDS),
    16, 17
sulphur compounds, airborne, 53, 54
Sweden
    Council of Environmental
        Information, 13
    dying lakes, 14, 42–5

2,4,5-T (2,4,5-trichlorophenoxyacetic
    acid), 33
TBT *see* tributyltin
teratogen, 22, 96
teratogenicity testing, 25
tetrachlorodibenzoparadioxin (TCDD),
    32
    see also dioxins
tetraethyl lead, 39, 97
Thames River, 49–50, 51, 63
thresholds, dose, 19, 25, 47
The Times, 21
Toxic Substances Control Act (ToSCA)
    1976 (USA), 28, 30
Toxic Substances Division, Department
    of Environment, 31
toxicokinetics, 97
toxicological testing, 10, 26
    genetic, 25, 26–7
    regulatory control, 29–30

trialkyltins, 31, 97
tributyltin (TBT), 31, 32, 97
    as antifouling agent, 31
trichlorophenol, 32
2,4,5-trichlorophenoxyacetic acid
    (2,4,5-T), 33
tsetse-fly control, 12
Tufts University, Boston, USA, 14
Turkey, 39, 41
typhus, 4, 8–9

UK
    acid rain from, 42–5
    air pollution, 45–8, 52–7, 59
    EU membership, 9
    strategy document on chemicals, 29
    water pollution, 49–51
ultraviolet (UV), 5, 71
UN *see* United Nations
UNECE *see* United Nations Economic
    Commission for Europe
UNEP *see* United Nations
    Environment Programme
Union Carbide India Limited, 34
United Nations (UN), 15
    Basel Convention (1989), 41
    Convention on the Law of the Sea
        (1982), 61, 62
United Nations Conference on the
    Human Environment, Stockholm
    (1972), 14, 42, 61, 62
United Nations Economic Commission
    for Europe (UNECE; ECE), 39, 44
United Nations Environment
    Programme (UNEP), 14, 39, 72
    International Register of Potentially
    Toxic Chemicals (IRPTC), 42
    Stockholm Convention (2001),
        39–41
universities, 32
USA
    influences on public opinion, 16

land use changes, 6
lead in petrol, 38
regulatory control, 28, 30

vanadium, 10
vanishing zero, 20
vector control, 12, 39
    see also malaria control
vegetarians, 22, 73
Venturi mask, 63, 97
Vietnam, 33
Villach, Austria, 15

Waldsterben, 44
waste
    in developing countries, 40
    dumping in sea, 58, 61, 62
    European regulations, 34, 59
    transfrontier movements, 41
    underground burial, 56, 59
    see also sewage
water pollution, 10, 45, 57–8, 60–6
    arsenic, 68
    buried waste, 56, 59
    effects of very low concentrations, 63–4
    health impact, 60–1, 63
    historical context, 3, 49–50
    legislation, 50
    nitrates, 20–1, 23, 51, 57–8
    nonagricultural sources, 61–2
    pesticides, 51, 56, 61–2
    Po Valley, Italy, 35
    research, 38
    see also marine pollution
Water Pollution Research Laboratory, 38
water quality, 50
    cost–benefit analysis, 21, 56
    EU standards, 20–1, 51, 56, 57–8, 65–6
    monitoring, 50–1
West Africa, 15
westerly winds, 43–4

wet chemical methods, 5
WHO (World Health Organization), 10
willingness-to-pay analysis, 55
WMO (World Meteorological
    Organization), 72
World Health Organization (WHO), 10
World Meteorological Organization
    (WMO), 72

xenotransplantation, 16, 97

zero tolerance, 6, 11–12, 20, 30

Index: Names

Biographical notes appear in bold

Ames, Bruce, 26, **89**
Aub, Joseph, 39

Bazalgette, Joseph, 63
Berry, Sir Colin, 6–7, 8–9, 11–12,
    15–17, 22–3, 25, 26, 30, 33, **89**
Booth, Sir Christopher, 67, **89**

Campbell, Moran, 63, **89**
Carson, Rachel, 3, 5, 6–7, 8, 12–14,
    19–20, 25, 26, 27, 31–2, 68, 69, 72,
    89–90
Carter, Richard, 13, 23, 25, 37, 48, 67,
    68–70, 71, **90**
Chadwick, Sir Edwin, 49, 63, 64
Condit, Celeste, 15–16
Corcoran, Peter, 7, 8, 10, 11, 29, 30,
    31, 37, 39–41, 61–2, **90**
Curry, Sir Donald, 62

Darwin, Charles, 18
Dayan, Anthony (Tony), 3, 6, 7, 8, 12,
    13, 14, 15, 17, 18–19, 22, 23–4, 25,
    26–7, 29–30, 31, 32, 34–5, 36,
    37–8, 40, 43–4, 45, 49, 52, 54,
    55–6, 60, 61, 62, 67, 69, 72, 73, **90**
Delaney, Thomas, 23–4
Des Voex, H A, 52
DeWitt, James, 11

Ehrlich, Paul, 7
Eldridge, Niles, 18
Evelyn, John, 52

Farman, Joseph (Joe), 28
Farmer, Peter, 18, 58, 59, 69, 71, **90–1**
Farr, William, 63

Flanagan, Robert, 20, 28, 31, 33, 46, **91**

Golding, Jean, 22
Gould, Stephen Jay, 18

Hamilton, Alice, 38
Howell, Dennis, 65
Hunter, Donald, 39, **91**
Hunter, Peter, 15, 28, 36, 39, 63, 64, **91**

Johnson, Stanley, 9–10, 20–1, 28, 30,
    33–4, 35, 37, 41–2, 44–5, 56–8,
    64–6, **91**

Kehoe, Robert, 38
Kilpatrick, Robert, 33

Lawther, Patrick (Pat), 36, 45–6, 47,
    48, **91**
Livingstone, Ken, 56, 60
Lovelock, James, 3–6, 8, 12–13, 17–18,
    21, 22, 27–8, 43, 54, 60, 71, 72–3, **91**

Macmillan, Harold (Lord Stockton), 53
Maynard, Robert (Bob), 23, 24–5, 35,
    36, 45–8, 52, 53, 54–5, 56, 59–60,
    63–4, 66–7, 69, 70, **92**
Mendel, Gregor, 18
Molina, Mario, 27
Müller, Paul, 4

Nabarro, Sir Gerald, 46, 53
Nixon, President Richard, 24

Palmlund, Ingar, 13–15, 42–3, 44, **92**

Ramazzini, Bernardino, 68
Reed, Leslie, 53, **92**
Rothschild, Lord, 27
Rowlands, Sherwood, 27
Russell, Bertrand (Lord Russell), 53
Russell, Earl John Francis Stanley
    (Frank), 53
Russell, Roland (Rollo), 53

Shore, Peter, 65
Simms, Dennis, 3, 10, 31, 37, 38, 43,
    52, 53, 54, 60–1, 62–3, 68, **92**
Smil, Vaclav, 6
Smith, Robert, 19–20, 26, 31–2, 66,
    71–2, **92**

Thomas, Keith, 12, 13
Thomas, Lewis, 4

Walker, Peter (The Rt. Hon.), 62
Waller, Robert, 52
Weber, Max, 9
Weighell, Sidney, 59–60
Williams, Richard Tecwyn, 19, **92–3**
Wilson, Edward, 72
Woods, Frank, 12, 17, 24, 35, 36,
    49–51, 56, 58, 64, **93**

Zeidler, Othmar, 4